Thyroid Ultrasonography and Fine Needle Aspiration Biopsy: A Practical Guide and Picture Atlas

Authored by

Samer El-Kaissi

Medical Subspecialties Institute, Endocrine Unit Cleveland Clinic Abu Dhabi, Al Maryah Island, Abu Dhabi, United Arab Emirates

&

Jack R Wall

The University of Sydney, The Bays Hospital, Mornington, Victoria, Australia

Thyroid Ultrasonography and Fine Needle Aspiration Biopsy: A Practical Guide and Picture Atlas

Authors: Samer El-Kaissi & Jack R Wall

ISBN (Online): 978-1-68108-685-9

ISBN (Print): 978-1-68108-755-9

Published by Bentham Science Publishers – Sharjah, UAE. All Rights Reserved.

First published in 2018.

General:

1. Any dispute or claim arising out of or in connection with this License Agreement or the Work (including non-contractual disputes or claims) will be governed by and construed in accordance with the laws of the U.A.E. as applied in the Emirate of Dubai. Each party agrees that the courts of the Emirate of Dubai shall have exclusive jurisdiction to settle any dispute or claim arising out of or in connection with this License Agreement or the Work (including non-contractual disputes or claims).
2. Your rights under this License Agreement will automatically terminate without notice and without the need for a court order if at any point you breach any terms of this License Agreement. In no event will any delay or failure by Bentham Science Publishers in enforcing your compliance with this License Agreement constitute a waiver of any of its rights.
3. You acknowledge that you have read this License Agreement, and agree to be bound by its terms and conditions. To the extent that any other terms and conditions presented on any website of Bentham Science Publishers conflict with, or are inconsistent with, the terms and conditions set out in this License Agreement, you acknowledge that the terms and conditions set out in this License Agreement shall prevail.

Bentham Science Publishers Ltd.
Executive Suite Y - 2
PO Box 7917, Saif Zone
Sharjah, U.A.E.
Email: subscriptions@benthamscience.org

BENTHAM SCIENCE

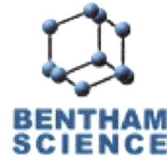

CONTENTS

PREFACE

Disorders of the thyroid and parathyroid glands are common and neck ultrasonography has stood the test of time and established itself as the primary imaging modality of not only the thyroid gland but also of the parathyroid glands and cervical lymph nodes. When clinically indicated, neck ultrasonography is invaluable and can be seen as an extension of the physical examination. It is performed in the office without any patient preparation and allows the physician to carry-out ultrasound-guided biopsies of anterior and lateral neck structures. Physicians who are not personally performing neck ultrasonography and ultrasound guided-procedures still need to be quite familiar with the ultrasound features of the normal and abnormal thyroid gland, parathyroid glands and cervical lymph nodes. This is particularly important as there is a wide variation in the standards of neck ultrasonography reporting.

The authors of this book are Endocrinologists with an interest in thyroid and parathyroid disorders, who have been performing neck ultrasonography and ultrasound-guided procedures of the neck for more than 15 years. When we set out to write this book, our aim was to provide a basic introduction to neck ultrasonography and to allow the reader to quickly search for relevant information about the ultrasound feature or condition in question. To aid with this task, we tried to include as many ultrasound images as possible and to limit the amount of text as we believe in the saying "a picture is worth a thousand words". This book would be a useful tool for endocrinologists, endocrine surgeons, cytopathologists, ultrasonographers and other health care workers with an interest in thyroid and parathyroid disorders. We would like to thank our family and friends who supported us with the writing of this book and hope that you enjoy it!

Samer El-Kaissi
Medical Subspecialties Institute,
Endocrine Unit Cleveland Clinic Abu Dhabi,
Al Maryah Island,
Abu Dhabi,
United Arab Emirates
E-mail: skaissi@hotmail.com

CHAPTER 1

Introduction to Thyroid Ultrasound

Abstract: Thyroid ultrasound has become an essential tool for the diagnosis of various thyroid disorders. It can be performed in the office during a medical consultation and is used to guide fine needle aspiration biopsies of the thyroid and cervical lymph nodes. Thyroid ultrasound waves are produced by piezoelectric crystals in response to electrical stimulation. These crystals also detect reflected incoming waves and produce a voltage that is used to construct an image. Beginning with A-mode imaging, thyroid ultrasound has evolved into inexpensive machines that produce high resolution two-dimensional B-images. Important properties of thyroid ultrasound waves that affect image quality and resolution include wavelength, propagation velocity, frequency, and acoustic impedance. Posterior shadowing, enhancement, and reverberation are common artefacts of neck ultrasonography and can be useful in defining certain features on ultrasound, such as posterior enhancement of cystic structures and the identification of colloid crystals in thyroid nodules due to reverberation. Colour Doppler and power Doppler help differentiate vascular structures in the neck, where power Doppler is more useful for smaller vessels.

Keywords: Acoustic impedance, Amplitude, Attenuation, B-mode ultrasound, Colour Doppler, Compound spatial imaging, Enhancement, Image resolution, Propagation velocity, Piezoelectric crystals, Posterior shadowing, Power Doppler, Reverberation, Refraction, Sound wave, Thyroid, Tissue harmonic imaging, Ultrasound, Ultrasound artefacts, Wavelength.

Since its first use in the 1960's, thyroid ultrasonography has become instrumental to the diagnosis and management of thyroid disorders. Thyroid ultrasound is particularly attractive because it is non-invasive, does not involve exposure to radiation and patient preparation is not required. The superficial location of the thyroid gland and other anatomical structures in the neck is ideal and allows the use of ultrasound-guided fine needle aspiration (FNA) to improve the diagnostic accuracy of thyroid ultrasound.

The reflection of sound waves from tissues that have different acoustic characteristics forms the basis of ultrasound imaging. Ultrasound waves are produced by piezoelectric crystals when stimulated by an electrical current.

Reflected sound waves are also detected by these crystals leading to the generation of a voltage.

Historically, ultrasound imaging started with A-mode imaging and an oscilloscope to detect reflected ultrasound waves. Subsequently, sequential A-mode images were aligned to produce two-dimensional cross-sectional images in what is known as B-mode ultrasound, although the images were grainy.

Todays' relatively inexpensive ultrasound machines produce clear, high resolution images. Tissue harmonic imaging (THI) and compound spatial imaging (CSI) have further enhanced the quality of ultrasound images, reducing noise and artefacts and allowing nodule definition with greater accuracy. THI uses integral multiples of the transmitted frequency to produce an image while CSI combines multiple images from different angles into a single image to eliminate scatter artefact [1, 2].

The basic characteristics of a sound wave are shown in Fig. (**1**). The trough of the sound wave is known as rarefaction while the point of peak pressure is referred to as compression. The distance from one compression point to the next is the wavelength (λ) and marks one cycle of the sound waves (Fig. **1**). The number of cycles per second is referred to as the frequency (f) of the wave and is measured in Hertz (Hz) so that one cycle per second is equivalent to 1 Hz. For neck ultrasound, high frequencies ranging from 7.5 to 15 megahertz (MHz) are used to image the relatively superficial structures of the neck. This is much higher than the audible sound frequency range of 20 – 20,000 Hz for humans. Amplitude is a measure of the intensity of the sound wave and a higher amplitude results in a brighter image on the monitor [1].

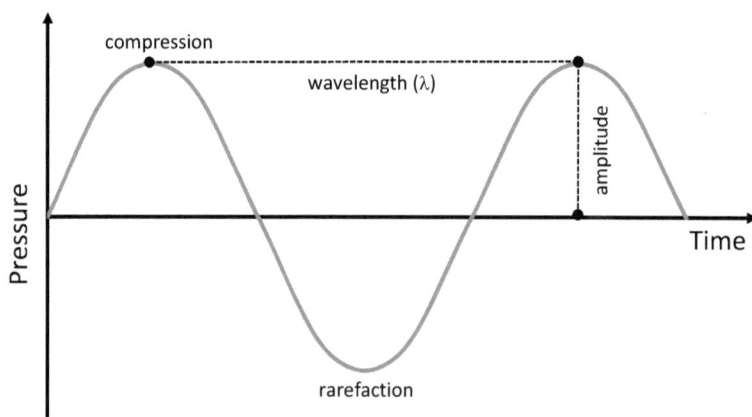

Fig. (1). Basic characteristics of a sound wave; λ = wavelength. Adapted from reference [1] with permission.

The propagation velocity (c), or speed of a sound wave, is a function of the wavelength and the frequency

$$c = f. \lambda$$

The propagation velocity is also influenced by the stiffness and density of the medium (Fig. **2**). It increases in a linear fashion with increasing stiffness of the medium and is inversely proportional to the density of the medium so that the propagation velocity through bone is much greater than that of air. The average propagation velocity of soft tissues is intermediate at 1540 m/sec [1], and is used to calculate distances where,

$$Distance = Time\ x\ Speed$$

As sound waves travel at a slightly lower speed in fatty tissues, distances can be underestimated in obese patients with increased fatty tissue in the neck.

The propagation velocity and the frequency of sound waves are important factors that impact image resolution. In order to discriminate between two points on ultrasound imaging, the wavelength should be less than or equal to the distance between these two points.

From the propagation velocity equation, It follows that the wavelength is directly related to the propagation velocity and inversely related to the frequency [1]

$$\lambda = \frac{c}{f}$$

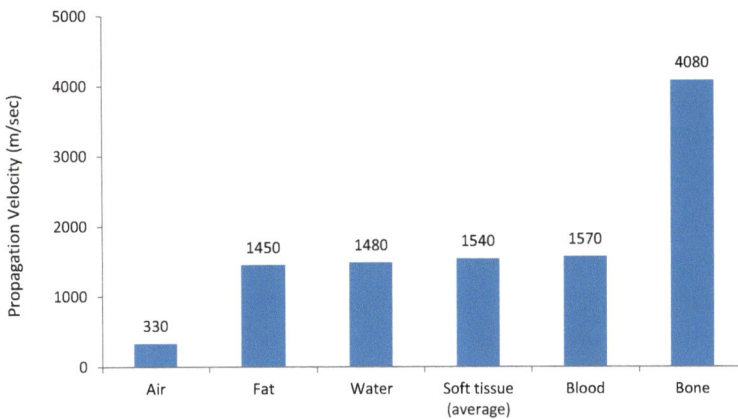

Fig. (2). Propagation velocity is influenced by the stiffness and density of the medium. Adapted from reference [1] with permission.

The propagation velocity impacts another important parameter, namely the acoustic impedance (Z), which is defined as the opposition that an ultrasound wave encounters when travelling through a particular medium. Acoustic impedance is directly proportional to the product of the propagation velocity and density of the medium (p), where

$$Z = p.c$$

The acoustic impedance of air is very low, that of soft tissue is intermediate while that of bone is very high. The greater the difference in acoustic impedance between different media, the greater the reflection of ultrasound waves. Ultrasound gel has a similar acoustic impedance to that of soft tissues, and its use as a coupling agent reduces ultrasound wave reflectance when imaging soft tissues [1].

Attenuation refers to the loss of sound wave energy due to scatter or due to absorption of sound waves by tissues and their conversion into heat. Many small anatomical structures in the neck scatter sound waves in different directions leading to grainy ultrasound images. These structures are known as diffuse reflectors, as opposed to specular reflectors such as the carotid artery and cystic structures which have smooth acoustic surfaces and reflect most of the sound waves much like a mirror, but at certain angles of imaging, they can deflect the waves away from the transducer leading to loss of signal.

Attenuation is greatest through air, followed by bone, soft tissues and is minimal through water. The higher the frequency of ultrasound, the greater the attenuation and the lower the tissue penetrance. Hence, high frequency ultrasound provides good resolution for superficial structures in the neck but would not be suitable for imaging deeper abdominal organs. For the latter, lower frequencies allow deeper penetration of ultrasound waves.

Ultrasound artefacts are common and include shadowing, enhancement, reverberation and refraction. While misleading at times, some artefacts can help define certain anatomical structures such as fluid-filled cysts and calcifications. Posterior shadowing refers to the loss of sound energy due to absorption as occurs in air or thick muscles, or due to the reflection of sound waves off calcified structures (Image **26**) and vessel walls (Image **1**). This leads to a hypoechoic shadow posterior to the imaged structure. In the case of a blood vessel wall, two dark lines may be seen and following these lines leads to the vessel (Image **1**). In contrast, enhancement of structures behind fluid-filled cavities (Image **4**) and blood vessels is due to the lower attenuation of fluids in relation to surrounding tissues [1, 3].

Reverberation refers to repeated reflection of the sound waves between two surfaces leading to the production of a ghost image. Reverberation accounts for the presence of multiple bright horizontal lines behind the trachea (Image **1**), the appearance of a solid-like component at the anterior margin of a cyst (Image **4**) and for the commonly seen comet tail sign of colloid crystals (Images **6** and **7**). The latter is due to the vibration of colloid crystals in response to ultrasound waves and this vibration is picked up by the transducer.

Refraction is the change in direction or the bending of ultrasound waves as they travel between two media with different propagation velocities. Refraction can alter the position of structures, although this phenomenon is not commonly seen in thyroid ultrasonography due to the superficial location of anatomical structures. Multipath artefacts are caused by specular reflectors and can lead to the appearance of a second false image, but this artefact is also uncommon in head and neck ultrasonography [1, 3].

When ultrasound waves bounce off a moving target, a change in wave frequency occurs and this is the basis for the Doppler effect [4]. Applying the Doppler effect to B-mode ultrasound images results in colour Doppler, which is often used to assess blood flow in head and neck ultrasonography. The intensity of Doppler frequency provides information about the relative velocity of blood flow and Doppler colour is indicative of the direction of flow, whereby red refers to flow towards the transducer and blue away from it.

Signal filtering is necessary for colour Doppler imaging to reduce the noise from operator movement and blood vessel pulsations. This leads to the exclusion of small blood vessels. Unlike colour Doppler, power Doppler integrates the total amount of flow and allows for imaging of the smaller blood vessels with increased signal-to-noise ratio, but does not provide information about the direction or velocity of flow. For this reason, power Doppler is most suitable for assessing the slower blood flow of smaller structures such as the cervical lymph nodes (CLNs).

For further reading on this topic, please see references [1 - 5].

CHAPTER 2

Anatomy of the Neck

Abstract: The thyroid gland is made up of two lobes joined by the isthmus and normally weighs approximately 30 grams. Embryologically, the gland develops from the endoderm at the floor of the pharynx and descends along the thyroglossal duct to the base of the anterior neck. The thyroglossal duct may fail to obliterate completely giving rise to thyroglossal duct cysts and may give rise to a small remnant known as the pyramidal lobe. In addition, ectopic thyroid tissue is commonly found along the thyroglossal duct path. There are normally four parathyroid glands, two superior glands located at the middle of the posterior border of the thyroid, and two inferior glands at the inferior border of the thyroid gland. However, there is some variability in the number and position of the parathyroid glands, especially the position of the inferior glands due to their embryologic origin. The normal parathyroid gland is too small to be seen on most imaging modalities including ultrasound. There are six cervical lymph node compartments of the anterior neck, labelled I to VI, including the retromanubrial compartment (also known as compartment VII) which is an extension of the central compartment (VI). The use of lymph node compartments during the ultrasound examination is essential for accurate localisation of cervical nodes in future ultrasound studies, to perform cervical node biopsies and for surgical excision of suspicious nodes.

Keywords: Carotid sheath, Cervical lymph nodes, Digastric muscle, Ectopic thyroid, Foramen caecum, Inferior thyroid artery, Internal jugular vein, Lingual thyroid, Pharynx, Pharyngeal pouches, Pyramidal lobe, Parathyroid, Sternocleidomastoid muscle, Strap muscles of the neck, Superior thyroid artery, Thyroid, Thyroglossal duct.

The thyroid gland is a butterfly-shaped organ made up of two lobes that normally extend from the thyroid cartilage down to the sixth tracheal ring. The left and right thyroid lobes are joined by the isthmus, a thin strip of thyroid tissue at the level of the second and third tracheal rings (Fig. **3**). The normal thyroid gland weighs around 30 grams with each lobe having the size of the distal phalanx of the thumb.

Samer El-Kaissi & Jack R Wall

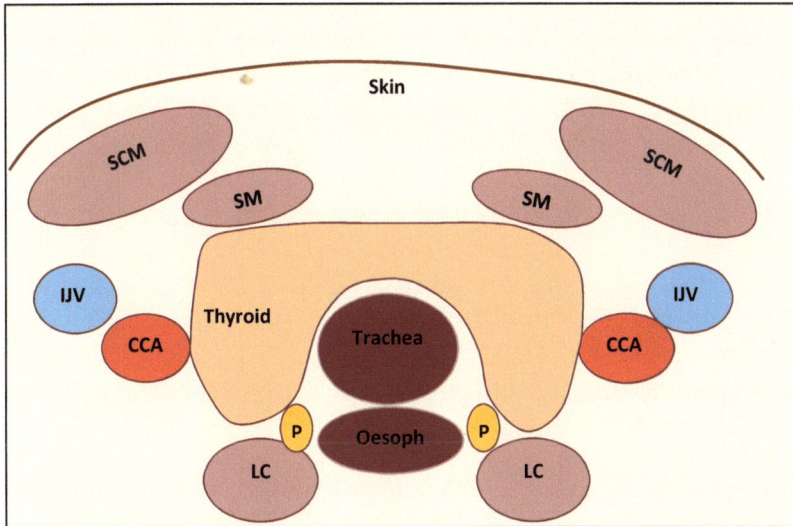

Fig. (3). Cross-sectional view of cervical viscera showing the relationship of the thyroid gland to the trachea, oesophagus and surrounding structures. LC: longus colli muscle, CCA: common carotid artery; IJV: internal jugular vein; SCM: sternocleidomastoid muscle; SM: strap muscles of the neck; P: parathyroid glands; Oesoph: oesophagus.

The thyroid gland develops from an endodermal thickening of the floor of the pharynx between the first and second pharyngeal pouches and migrates caudally into the neck along the thyroglossal duct (TGD). Ectopic thyroid tissue can occur along the TGD path and is most commonly seen at the foramen caecum at the base of the tongue, known as *lingual thyroid*. Up to two-thirds of patients with a lingual thyroid do not have any other thyroid tissue. Less commonly, ectopic thyroid tissue may be seen in the mediastinum, oesophagus or heart.

The pyramidal lobe is a small remnant of the TGD most commonly seen projecting superiorly from the left isthmus, particularly in patients with Graves' disease. Failure of the TGD to obliterate completely after the descent of the thyroid gland leads to the development of TGD cysts (Image **20**). Ectopic thyroid tissue and TGD cysts are occasionally affected by thyroid cancer, making their identification and evaluation of clinical relevance.

Blood supply to the thyroid gland is from the superior thyroid artery, a branch of the external carotid artery, and the inferior thyroid artery which branches from the thyrocervical trunk that in turn branches off the subclavian artery. Venous drainage of the thyroid gland is *via* the thyroid veins into the internal jugular and innominate veins.

The parathyroid glands are located posterior to the thyroid gland. There are usually four parathyroid glands, two superior and two inferior glands, but the number can vary from two to six glands. The superior glands are located at the middle of the posterior border of the thyroid, while the inferior glands are usually at the inferior border of the thyroid. Because of their embryonic origin, the position of the inferior parathyroids is more variable than the superior glands, and they may be located in the superior mediastinum, retro-oesophageal space, and rarely intrathyroidal. The superior and inferior thyroid arteries provide vascular supply to the superior and inferior parathyroid glands, respectively. Venous drainage is into the thyroid veins. Normal parathyroid glands have a flattened oval-shaped appearance and are too small to be seen on most imaging modalities, measuring around 6 x 4 mm or less.

The neck houses over 300 CLNs which may become enlarged in inflammatory, infectious or malignant conditions. The sternocleidomastoid muscle divides the neck into anterior and posterior triangles, which can be further subdivided into the following lymph node compartments (Fig. **4**):

I. Extends anteriorly from the posterior edge of the submandibular glands. It is bounded superiorly by the mandible and inferiorly by the hyoid bone, and is divided into submental (IA) and submandibular (IB) compartments by the anterior belly of the digastric muscle.

II. Extends from the anterior border of the carotid sheath to the posterior border of the sternocleidomastoid muscle. It is bounded superiorly by the mandible and inferiorly by the level of the hyoid bone. This compartment may be further subdivided by the anterior border of the sternocleidomastoid muscle into IIA anteriorly and IIB posteriorly.

III. Extends from the anterior border of the carotid sheath to the posterior border of the sternocleidomastoid muscle. It is bounded superiorly by the level of the hyoid bone and inferiorly by the level of the cricoid cartilage.

IV. Extends from the anterior border of the carotid sheath to the posterior border of the sternocleidomastoid muscle. It is bounded superiorly by the level of the cricoid cartilage and inferiorly by the clavicle.

V. Extends from the posterior border of the sternocleidomastoid muscle to the anterior border of the trapezius muscle. It is bounded superiorly by the occipital process and inferiorly by the clavicle, and can be subdivided into VA superiorly and VB inferiorly by the level of the cricoid cartilage.

VI. Extends from the anterior border of the carotid sheaths and is bounded superiorly by the hyoid bone, inferiorly by the brachiocephalic (innominate) artery and houses the thyroid gland.

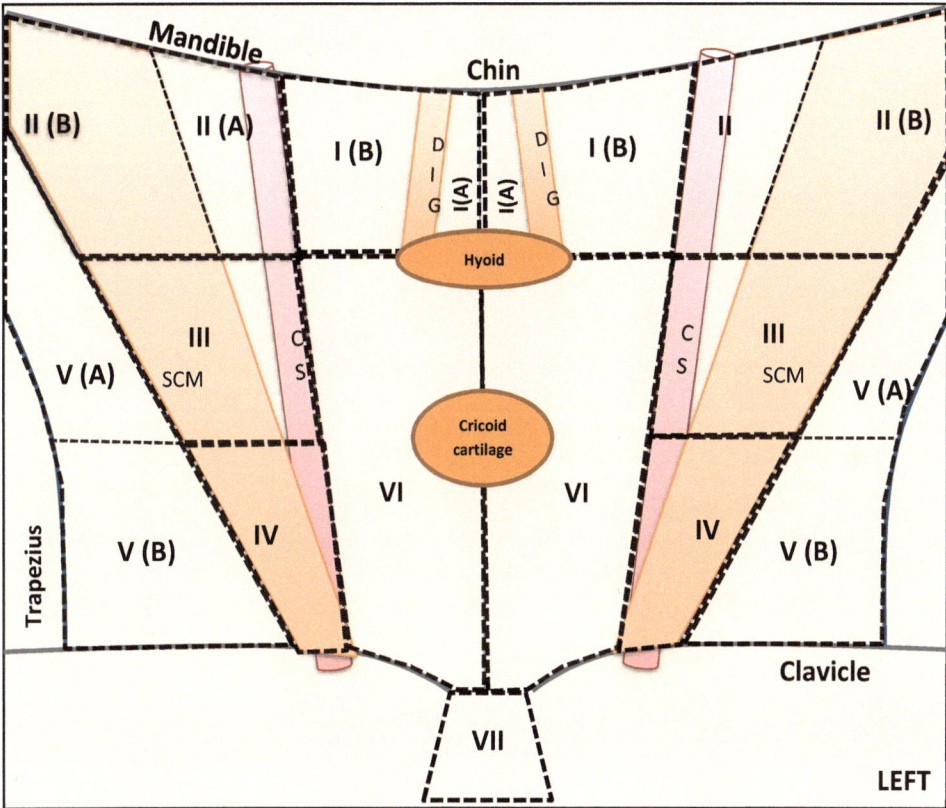

Fig. (4). Lymph node compartments of the anterior neck. DIG – anterior belly of the digastric muscle, CS – carotid sheath, SCM – sternocleidomastoid muscle.

In addition, the space behind the manubrium just below the suprasternal notch is an extension of the central compartment (VI) and is referred to as compartment VII. It houses the pretracheal and paratracheal lymph nodes that may be affected in thyroid disease. This compartment can be viewed during ultrasound examination of the neck by angling the probe inferiorly.

For further reading on this topic, please see references [6, 7].

CHAPTER 3

Ultrasound of the Normal Thyroid Gland

Abstract: Thyroid ultrasound is used in clinical practice to assess thyroid gland volume and vascularity, assess thyroid nodules and cervical lymph nodes, examine the parathyroid glands in patients with primary hyperparathyroidism, guide biopsies, aspiration and ablation of thyroid and anterior neck structures, and in post-operative thyroid cancer surveillance. However, thyroid ultrasound is not suitable as a screening tool of the thyroid. Ultrasound examination of the thyroid follows a systematic approach beginning with the thyroid gland volume, echogenicity, echotexture, Doppler flow and a detailed examination of any thyroid nodules. This is followed by an examination of the anterior neck cervical lymph nodes, and the parathyroid glands if clinically indicated. The normal thyroid gland is echogenic compared to the neck muscles and displays little or no vascularity on Doppler study. The size of a normal thyroid gland is 4-6 cm in length, 1.3-1.8 cm anteroposteriorly, and the isthmus width is less than 6 mm. The thyroid ultrasound report should provide information about the examination technique, a brief summary of the indications for the ultrasound, detailed findings of the examination, conclusions and management recommendations.

Keywords: Cervical lymph nodes, Doppler, Echogenicity, Echotexture, Indications, Microbubble contrast, Margins, Nodule, Retrosternal goitre, Thyroid, Thyroid ultrasound reporting, Thyroid volume, Transducer, Ultrasound, Ultrasound elastography.

Ultrasound imaging of the thyroid gland and anterior neck is an extremely sensitive tool that allows detection of thyroid nodules as small as 2 mm, assessment of CLNs and parathyroid glands. Common indications for thyroid and anterior neck ultrasonography include [8]:

1. Evaluation of clinically palpable thyroid nodules or CLNs to assess size and ultrasound characteristics, and whether FNA biopsy is indicated
2. Evaluation of patients with goitre to objectively determine the thyroid gland volume and exclude nodular disease
3. Examination of the thyroid gland in patients with an equivocal clinical examination

4. Screening for malignancy of the thyroid gland in high risk patients such as those with a history of radiation exposure, familial forms of differentiated thyroid cancer or history of cancer syndromes in first-degree relatives *e.g.* Cowden's disease, Carney's complex, Werner syndrome and multiple endocrine neoplasia 2A (MEN 2A)
5. Detection of parathyroid adenoma in patients with primary hyperparathyroidism
6. Pre-operative assessment of the thyroid gland and CLNs in patients with thyroid cancer
7. Post-operative thyroid cancer surveillance, looking for residual thyroid tissue, recurrent disease and cervical lymphadenopathy
8. Ultrasound-guided FNA biopsies of thyroid nodules, parathyroid adenomas and CLNs
9. Ultrasound-guided alcohol sclerotherapy, radiofrequency or laser ablation of thyroid nodules and CLNs
10. Monitoring of previously identified thyroid nodules, parathyroid adenomas or CLNs
11. Doppler flow examination of the thyroid in patients with hyperthyroidism to help differentiate thyroiditis from Graves' disease.

While ultrasound of the thyroid is extremely useful and sensitive for the detection of thyroid nodules, it should not be used to screen patients outside the indications listed above as this may lead to over-diagnosis of thyroid nodules, unnecessary tests and patient anxiety.

After explaining the procedure to the patient, the patient is placed in a supine position and the neck is extended by placing a pillow behind the shoulders. The degree of neck extension may be limited in patients with osteoarthritis of the cervical spine so that the position of the pillow should be adjusted to keep the patient as comfortable as possible. It is preferable to have the ultrasound monitor facing the physician or above the patient's head so that the physician does not need to look away from the patient during the procedure. Acoustic gel serves as a coupling agent and is applied to the foot of a linear-array transducer. The superficial location of the thyroid gland and its surrounding structures in the neck allows the use of a high frequency transducer (12-15 MHz) which increases the ability to detect nodules two-fold when compared to a 7.5 MHz transducer [9]. Examination of the thyroid is performed in a systematic fashion in the transverse and longitudinal views, beginning with a scout view of the whole gland, then the isthmus, followed by each of the left and right lobes, assessment of the anterior cervical nodes and finally the parathyroid glands if clinically indicated.

On ultrasound, the normal thyroid gland has a fine homogeneous echogenic 'sandy' appearance with a bright hyperechoic capsule (Image **1**). The sternocleidomastoid and strap muscles of the neck (sternothyroid and sternohyoid) are hypoechoic compared to the thyroid gland while the surrounding fascia of the muscle is hyperechoic. The carotid artery lies medial to the jugular vein and both structures are anechoic with posterior enhancement but unlike the jugular vein, the carotid artery is pulsatile and non-compressible. The trachea is a hypoechoic structure located centrally behind the isthmus and surrounded on either side by the thyroid lobes. Its reverberation artefact appears as multiple echogenic rings on ultrasound. The oesophagus is normally tucked behind the left thyroid lobe and has a hypoechoic muscular rim with an echogenic centre giving it the appearance of a bull's eye (Image **3**). It can be seen dilate during swallowing.

The normal thyroid gland measures 4-6 cm in length and 1.3-1.8 cm antero-posteriorly. The isthmus thickness is 4-6 mm. The average volume (± standard deviation) of the normal thyroid gland is 18.6 ± 4.5 cc and is usually smaller in females (17.5 ± 4.2) compared to males (19.6 ± 4.7) [10, 11]. The volume of the thyroid gland is estimated by adding the volumes of the left and right lobes, which in turn are calculated from their respective dimensions (in cm) as follows:

$$\textit{Volume of thyroid lobe (cc)} = \textit{Length x Width x Depth x } \frac{\pi}{6}$$

Respective synonyms for the three dimensions include height, transverse and anteroposterior (AP) diameters. Most ultrasound machines calculate the lobe volumes automatically once the dimensions are entered. In patients with large goitres where the gland dimensions may exceed the width of the foot of the transducer, switching to a low frequency curved (abdominal) transducer or using the panoramic function if available, allows capture of the whole lobe on the screen.

Assessment of gland vascularity with colour Doppler may be useful in discerning Graves' disease from other conditions such as thyroiditis [12]. The normal thyroid gland has minimal vascularity (Images **2** and **3**). In Graves' disease, Doppler flow is markedly increased throughout the gland during the active phase of the illness, known as 'thyroid inferno' (Image **49**). The Doppler flow correlates with the degree of hyperthyroidism and decreases gradually as euthyroidism is restored [13] (Image **51**). A peak systolic velocity greater than 60 cm/sec [normal 15-30 cm/sec] in the inferior thyroid artery has been reported to be highly specific for Graves' disease [14]. In Hashimoto's thyroiditis, Doppler study of the thyroid is less helpful as it may be increased, decreased or normal (Image **56**). In Amiodarone-induced hyperthyroidism (AIH), Doppler flow is increased in type 1 AIH and reduced or absent in type 2 AIH.

Because Doppler imaging does not provide information about capillary blood flow, microbubble contrast agents have been developed. These are injected intravenously and the 3-5 micron air bubbles reflect sound waves thereby allowing visualization of small capillaries. The role of microbubble contrast in the evaluation of thyroid nodules [15] and cervical nodes [16] remains to be determined.

It may be possible to partially view retrosternal goitres with the neck in the extended position by having the patient swallow. Tilting the probe caudally will also allow visualization of cervical lymph nodes in the substernal space (compartment VII). The pyramidal lobe is present in about 80% of people but is not commonly seen on ultrasound because of its small size, although it may be visibly enlarged in patients with Graves' disease. Similarly, normal parathyroid glands are small and not usually seen on ultrasound examination.

At the end of the examination, a detailed report is generated noting thyroid size, echogenicity, echotexture, vascularity, and describing any nodules or cervical nodes. The report should also provide a comparison with previous ultrasound examinations, if available, and a concise conclusion with treatment and follow-up recommendations (Table **1**).

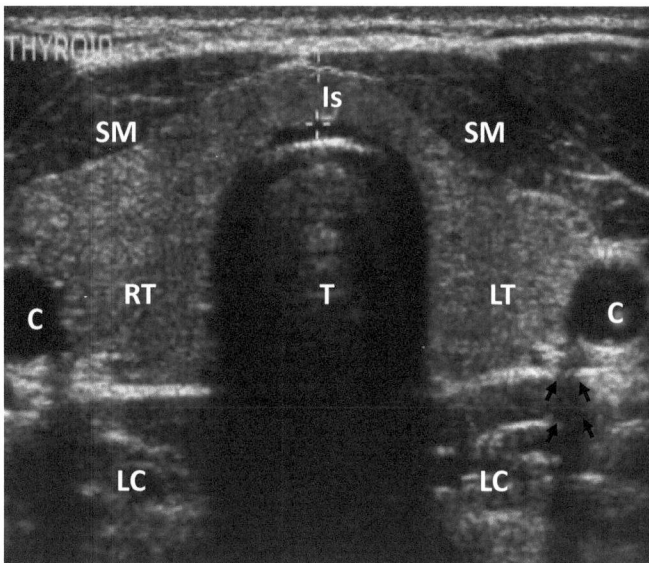

Image (1). Normal thyroid sonogram, transverse view. The gland appears hyperechoic in relation to the strap muscles of the neck (SM). Notice the hypoechoic shadow (black arrows) posterior to the left common carotid artery (C) due to the reflection of sound waves. The bright horizontal lines in the trachea (T) are due to a reverberation artefact. Longus colli muscle (LC), right thyroid lobe, (RT), left thyroid lobe (LT), isthmus (Is).

Table 1. Thyroid ultrasound standardized reporting. US – ultrasound; USE – ultrasound elastography. Adapted from reference [17] with permission.

US Report subheading	Description
Technique	➢ US equipment
	➢ Probe
	➢ Patient with compromising factors *e.g.* restricted neck extension
Clinical details	➢ Clinical indication for thyroid US scan
	➢ Clinical risk factors for thyroid cancer including family or personal history of thyroid cancer
	➢ Previous thyroid or neck surgery
	➢ Previous FNA results
Results	➢ Thyroid dimensions x3 and volume (right and left lobes)
	➢ Isthmus width (transverse view)
	➢ Echogenicity and vascularity of the thyroid gland
	➢ Echotexture of the gland (homogeneous or heterogeneous)
	➢ Nodules
	o Laterality: left lobe, right lobe or isthmus
	o Location: superior, middle or inferior
	o Size in 3 dimensions ± volume
	o Shape
	o Margins:
	▪ Well defined and smooth
	▪ Ill-defined
	▪ Irregular (infiltrative, lobulated or spiculated)
	o Echotexture (homogeneous or heterogeneous)
	o Echogenicity if homogeneous echotexture (hypoechoic, isoechoic or hyperechoic)
	o Composition
	o Echogenic foci
	o Extrathyroidal extension
	o USE, if available
	o Change in size from the previous examination
	o Risk of malignancy
	o Whether FNA biopsy is indicated
	➢ Retrosternal extension and/or tracheal deviation
	➢ Cervical lymph nodes (levels I-VII)
	o Location
	o Size (short axis and long axis, 3 dimensions if size > 1 cm)
	o Shape
	o Echogenicity
	o Fatty hilum: present or absent
	o Vascularity: normal (central) or peripheral
	o High suspicion features such as cystic aspect, microcalcifications, hyperechoic component
Conclusion	➢ Normal examination or type of pathology
	➢ Comparison to previous US scans
	➢ Management and follow-up recommendations

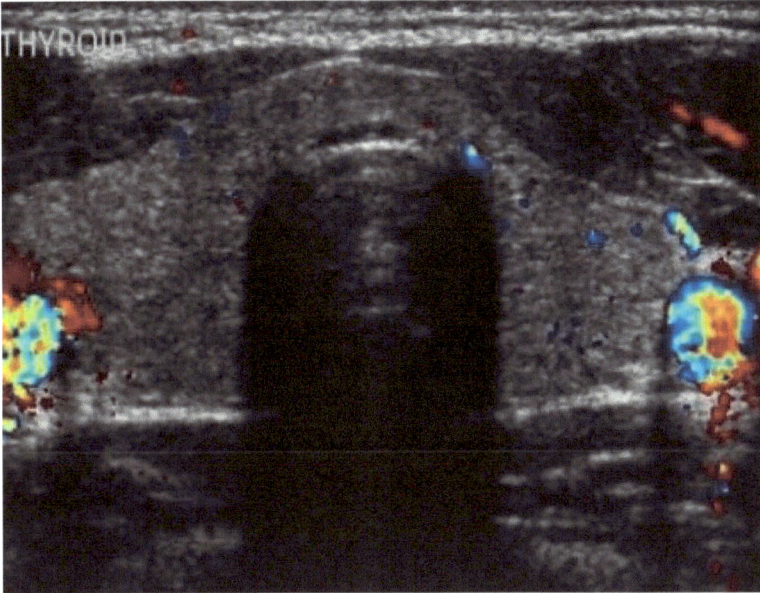

Image (2). Normal thyroid Doppler study displaying minimal flow in the thyroid gland.

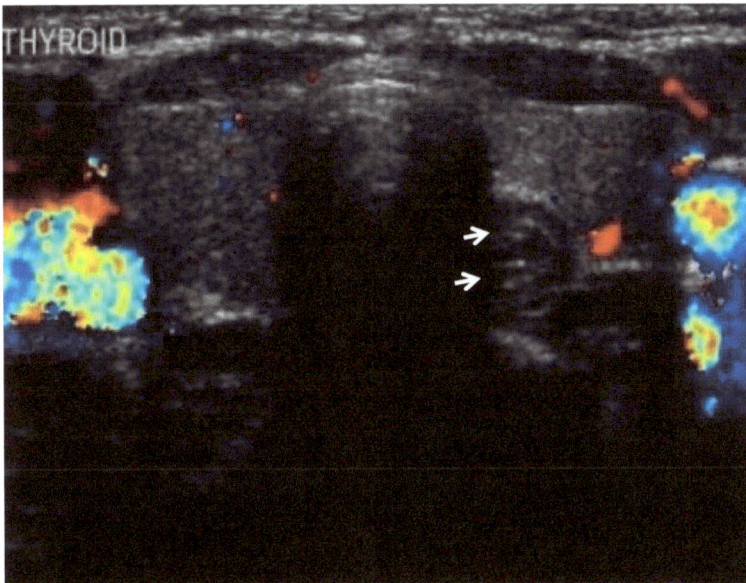

Image (3). Normal thyroid Doppler study with minimal flow in the thyroid gland. The oesophagus can be seen at the postero-medial border of the left lobe (arrows).

CHAPTER 4

Ultrasound of Nodular Thyroid Disease

Abstract: Thyroid ultrasound examination allows detailed and accurate description of thyroid nodule features including nodule size, location, echotexture, echogenicity, margins, shape, presence and extent of cystic content, calcifications, and nodular flow pattern on Doppler study. The finding of a colloid signal, complete thin peripheral halo, or complete rim calcification makes thyroid nodule malignancy less likely, whereas nodule hypoechogenicity, microcalcifications, irregular margins, taller than wide shape, and interrupted rim calcification with extrusion of soft tissue are suggestive of malignancy. In contrast to papillary thyroid carcinoma, follicular thyroid carcinoma does not display microcalcifications or cystic content on ultrasound, often has a regular margin and may feature a peripheral halo. The role of ultrasound elastography and Doppler flow in distinguishing benign from malignant nodules remains to be determined. Importantly, no single ultrasound feature in isolation is predictive of nodule malignancy or benignancy, and the risk of malignancy is best characterised using a combination of ultrasound features. Two widely used thyroid malignancy risk stratification systems are the American Thyroid Association and the European Thyroid Imaging Reporting and Data System. These classification systems improve the sensitivity of ultrasound for the detection of thyroid malignancy without compromising its specificity and allow the recommendation of nodule size cut-offs for FNA biopsy.

Keywords: Anaplastic thyroid carcinoma, Colloid, Differentiated thyroid cancer, European Thyroid Imaging Reporting and Data System, Follicular thyroid carcinoma, Hypoechoic, Thyroid, Nodule, Ultrasound, Multinodular goitre, Retrosternal goitre, Papillary thyroid carcinoma, Medullary thyroid carcinoma, Microcalcifications, Rim calcification, Taller-than-wide, Spongiform, Peripheral halo.

A thyroid nodule is a discrete thyroid lesion that can be distinguished by ultrasound from surrounding thyroid tissue. Clinically palpable thyroid nodules occur in approximately 5% of women and 1% of men [18], although on thyroid ultrasound examination up to 68% of adults are found to have thyroid nodules [9]. Furthermore, among patients with a palpable thyroid nodule who were referred for ultrasonography, 48% had additional nodules [19]. These findings are supported by autopsy studies suggesting that up to 50% of patients with no clinical evidence of thyroid nodularity had at least one thyroid nodule, one-third of which were greater than 2 cm [20].

Samer El-Kaissi & Jack R Wall

The estimated risk of malignancy in a thyroid nodule is around 7-15% [21, 22], and is similar in patients with palpable and those with non-palpable or incidental nodules [23]. The risk of thyroid malignancy in multinodular goitre (MNG) is similar to that of solitary thyroid nodules [24] so that the risk of malignancy per nodule decreases as the number of nodules increases [25]. The size of a thyroid nodule does not help to distinguish benign from malignant disease and assessing only the dominant nodule in a MNG should be avoided as non-dominant malignant nodules may be missed in up to 30% of cases [26]. Each nodule should be assessed individually with ultrasound and if malignancy is suspected, FNA biopsy can be considered. In Large goitres with retrosternal extension, tilting the transducer caudally while the patient swallows allow a glimpse of the retrosternal thyroid. If clinically indicated, further imaging of a retrosternal goitre with endoscopic ultrasonography, computed tomography (CT) or magnetic resonance imaging (MRI) may be performed. Endoscopic ultrasonography is particularly advantageous because FNA biopsies can be performed on retrosternal nodules during the scan.

There are 3 main types of thyroid cancer, namely differentiated thyroid cancer (DTC), medullary thyroid carcinoma (MTC) and anaplastic thyroid carcinoma. DTC comprises more than 90% of all thyroid malignancies [27] and includes papillary (PTC) and follicular (FTC) thyroid cancer. PTC makes up 80-85% of all thyroid cancers, is twice as common in women as it is in men and peaks in the third and fourth decades of life. While multifocal PTC's and CLN involvement are not uncommon, distant metastases occur less frequently and are more common in aggressive variants such as tall-cell, columnar and hobnail PTC. PTC presents on ultrasound as a solid hypoechoic lesion that may be associated with microcalcifications, irregular margins, a predominance of central vascularity, and CLN involvement. Importantly, up to 5% of mixed nodules harbour malignancy [28] and of all PTCs, up to 26% occur in mixed nodules [29, 30]. The follicular variant of PTC displays similar features to FTC on ultrasound (Image **35**).

FTC makes up 5-10% of thyroid cancers. It is three times more common in women as in men with a peak incidence in the fifth decade of life. Compared to PTC, vascular invasion, haematogenous spread and distant metastatic disease are more common. However, distant metastases are rarely seen in tumours smaller than 2 cm [31]. On ultrasound, FTC appears as a slightly hypoechoic, isoechoic or hyperechoic homogeneous lesion with regular margins and occasionally a peripheral halo representing a thin capsule. The tumour may be oval-shaped, cuboidal or taller than wide, and may display increased central vascularity but microcalcifications and cystic components are uncommon. Hurthle cell lesions, 20% of which are malignant, are a subtype of FTC with a similar appearance on ultrasound.

MTC arises from the parafollicular C-cells and makes up 2-5% of thyroid malignancies. Up to one-third of cases are associated with multiple endocrine neoplasia 2A or 2B, and the remaining two-thirds of cases are sporadic. The disease affects an equal number of men and women, and commonly spreads to the cervical lymph nodes and distally. On ultrasound (Image **34**), MTC appears as a solid hypoechoic lesion, often with increased central vascularity and hyperechoic foci, representing amyloid deposition and calcifications [32].

Anaplastic thyroid carcinoma, thyroid lymphoma arising in the setting of chronic Hashimoto's thyroiditis and involvement of the thyroid in non-thyroidal metastatic disease are much less common, accounting for less than 5% of all thyroid malignancies.

The annual incidence of thyroid carcinoma in the United States has almost tripled over the past 3 decades, jumping from 4.9 cases per 100,000 in 1975 to 14.3 cases per 100,000 in 2009, with PTC registering the greatest increase [33]. While it is argued that the use of sensitive ultrasound imaging has contributed to this increase through the detection of non-palpable thyroid nodules, other factors are likely to be involved as only half of the increased thyroid cancer incidence is due to microcarcinomas ($\leq$ 1 cm), with malignancies measuring 1.1-2.0 cm (30%) and greater than 2.0 cm (20%) making up the other-half [34]. Despite the increasing incidence, there has been no change in the low mortality rate of thyroid cancer, approximately 0.5 deaths per 100,000 [33].

Assessment of thyroid nodules with ultrasound is performed in a systematic fashion as described in Table **1**. After noting the location of the nodule, its 3 dimensions $\pm$ volume are measured. Nodules with a peripheral halo should be measured with the callipers placed on the outer edge of the halo. For subcentimetric nodules (< 1 cm), measurement of the largest dimension (usually its length) and AP diameter are sufficient.

Subsequently, a thorough assessment of the nodule's ultrasound characteristics is performed [17, 35]:

1. Echotexture:
   a. Homogeneous: uniform echogenicity throughout the nodule
   b. Heterogeneous: mixed hypoechoic and isoechoic components within the nodule (Images **17** and **24**)
2. Echogenicity of homogeneous nodules is compared to the surrounding thyroid tissue. In patients with suspected Hashimoto's thyroiditis, a comparison in relation to the submandibular glands may be more accurate. Echogenicity can be classified as follows:
   a. Hypoechoic: nodule echogenicity is less than that of the surrounding

thyroid parenchyma (Images **21-23** and **25**). The European Thyroid Association (ETA) guidelines define such nodules as 'mildly hypoechoic' and those with lower echogenicity compared to the strap muscles as 'markedly hypoechoic' [17]

    b. Isoechoic: nodule echogenicity is similar to that of the surrounding thyroid parenchyma (Image **18**)

    c. Hyperechoic: nodule echogenicity is greater than that of the surrounding thyroid parenchyma (Images **58** and **59**)

3. Shape of the nodule [17]:

    a. Oval: AP diameter to transverse diameter ratio < 1 and AP diameter to height ratio < 1 in the transverse and longitudinal planes, respectively

    b. Round: AP diameter to transverse diameter ratio = 1 and AP diameter to height ratio = 1 in the transverse and longitudinal planes, respectively

    c. Taller-than-wide (TTW): AP diameter to transverse diameter ratio > 1 in the transverse plane (Images **31** and **32**)

    d. Taller-than-long: AP diameter to height ratio > 1 in the longitudinal plane

4. Character of the nodule (Fig. **5**): solid, mixed (complex), cystic or spongiform. The extent of the cystic component due to degeneration, colloid deposition or a previous haemorrhage can be visually approximated as follows [17]:

    a. Solid or predominantly solid (< 10% cystic)

    b. Mixed predominantly solid (10-50% cystic, Image **15**)

    c. Mixed predominantly cystic (50-90% cystic, Images **9-14**)

    d. Cystic (> 90% cystic, Image **8**). Pure cysts (Images **4** and **27**) without wall thickening and no solid component are uncommon making up less than 2% of all thyroid nodules. They are classified as benign nodules [36 - 38].

    e. Spongiform nodules contain multiple tiny cysts occupying the entire nodule (Image **5**). Colloid crystals and echogenic enhancement of the posterior wall of microcysts are often seen on ultrasound. Spongiform nodules have a very low suspicion for thyroid malignancy ≤ 3% [17, 39]

5. Nodule margins [35]: definition and regularity. Unlike irregular margins, ill-defined margins lack clear demarcation from the surrounding thyroid tissue (Images **34** and **36**) and may be seen in both benign and malignant nodules. On the other hand, irregular margins are associated with thyroid malignancy and can be further subclassified as:

    a. Infiltrative: irregular margin without spiculations or microlobulations (Images **28** and **33**)

    b. Microlobulated: one or more smooth round protrusions of the nodule margin (Image **29**)

    c. Spiculated: one or more sharp spike-like protrusions of the margin (Image **30**)

6. Presence of calcification and its nature. Two types of calcifications are

described in thyroid nodules, namely microcalcification and macrocalcification.

    a. Microcalcification refers to punctate (≤ 1 mm) specks of calcium deposits without acoustic shadowing (Images **31-33**). They are often associated with PTC and probably represent psammoma bodies, and rarely in MTC (Image **34**) due to calcified amyloid deposits [40]. Occasionally, microcalcifications in PTC may coalesce in an appearance similar to macrocalcifications with an acoustic shadow [41].

    b. Macrocacifications present as larger (> 1 mm) dense calcifications with an acoustic shadow and are often due to tissue necrosis. They may occur as intra-nodular macrocalcifications or present on the periphery of a nodule in what is described as rim or 'eggshell' calcification (Images **19** and **23**). Intra-nodular macrocalcifications of the entire nodule carry a low risk of malignancy [17], whereas short echogenic line calcifications may be seen in both benign and malignant nodules and are not consistently associated with thyroid malignancy [42]. Continuous rim calcification of a thyroid nodule suggests benignancy, whereas incomplete rim calcification (Image **27**) with extrusion of thyroid (tumour) tissue is suggestive of malignancy [43]. Importantly, complete rim calcification may not be fully appreciated on ultrasound due to acoustic shadowing (Image **26**).

7. Doppler study depicting nodular blood flow distribution and intensity. Thyroid nodule Doppler flow can be classified into 3 grades [17, 44]:

    a. Grade I: no visible flow

    b. Grade II: peripheral flow ± slight intra-nodular flow covering less than 50% of the nodule area (Images **15**, **16**, **18**, **24** and **25**)

    c. Grade III: marked intra-nodular flow covering 50% or more of the nodule area ± slight peripheral flow (Images **17** and **23**)

Doppler flow can be used for better definition of ill-defined nodules (Image **25**) and in mixed nodules it helps to differentiate solid tissue from colloid and fibrin deposits [17]. Intranodular flow may be associated with an increased risk of thyroid malignancy, although the ability of Doppler flow to discriminate benign from malignant nodules has been questioned with some studies suggesting that Doppler flow is beneficial [23, 29, 45, 46] but not other studies [47 - 50]. While central vascularity is seen in up to 74% of malignant nodules, peripheral vascularity has been documented in 22% of malignant nodules thereby reducing the specificity of this feature for diagnosing malignancy [29]. Therefore, intra-nodular flow on Doppler may not provide any additional benefits over grey-scale features in PTC [51] and may be more useful for the diagnosis of FTC [23, 36, 52]. In one study, the use of a 5-grade Doppler classification system improved the sensitivity and specificity of thyroid cancer detection [53].

Ultrasound elastography (USE) is a technique that estimates tissue elasticity and may be useful in determining the malignant potential of thyroid nodules. USE measures the distortion of a thyroid nodule to external pressure applied with the transducer (strain elastography), or to internal strain from the pulsating carotid artery (shear-wave elastography). A number of USE scoring systems are available, of which the strain index is very informative as it compares thyroid nodule strain to that of normal thyroid tissue [54]. In clinical practice, a meta-analysis of more than 600 thyroid nodules showed that USE has a high sensitivity (92%) and specificity (90%) for the detection of malignant thyroid nodules [55]. In a prospective study of more than 900 thyroid nodules, USE had a high sensitivity with a robust negative predictive value (NPV) at 97% although the positive predictive value (PPV) was poor at 36% [56]. USE may have a role in reducing the number of FNA biopsies in low-risk thyroid nodules [57] and in averting diagnostic thyroidectomy in patients with indeterminate thyroid nodules on FNA [58], but should not replace a greyscale ultrasound study. Major limitations of USE is that it has a high inter-observer variability [59] and cannot be used on thyroid nodules with egg-shell or macrocalcification, complex nodules with a cystic component exceeding 25% of the nodule volume, large nodules > 3 cm, nodules located posteriorly or in the isthmus, or in multinodular goitres where the thyroid nodules are confluent and not easily distinguishable from one another [11, 17].

During the examination, the sonographer is actively looking for features that help to differentiate benign from malignant nodules (Table **2**). Benign features include the presence of a peripheral halo (Images **10** and **15**) around the nodule, a spongiform nodule (Image **5**), and a colloid signal (Images **6** and **7**) [35]. The latter presents on ultrasound as echogenic colloid crystals with a posterior reverberation artefact known as a comet tail or ring-down artefact. Occasionally, colloid can be seen as a larger 'colloid clot' with a honeycomb pattern [60]. In mixed nodules, we sometimes encounter hyperechoic deposits (Image **8**) of unknown clinical significance [17]. These deposits often lack significant flow on Doppler study and may represent debris or haemorrhage. A peripheral halo corresponds to a nodular capsule and compressed thyroid tissue and blood vessels. Although a complete thin halo predicts benignancy with a specificity of 95%, a halo is absent in more than half of benign nodules and may be present in up to 24% of malignant nodules [61 - 63]. A thicker than usual halo has also been associated with thyroid malignancy, especially the follicular variant of PTC (Image **35**) and FTC [17]. It is therefore important to assess all the ultrasonographic features of a nodule to determine its risk of malignancy.

Potential features of malignancy (mostly PTC) on ultrasound include a solid hypoechoic nodule (Images **21-23** and **25**) or solid hypoechoic component of a complex nodule that may be associated with one or more of the following features: irregular margins (Images **28** and **30**), taller-than-wide shape (Images **31** and **32**), microcalcifications (Images **31-33**), interrupted rim calcifications with soft tissue extrusion, or suspicious cervical lymphadenopathy. The risk of malignancy in these nodules exceeds 70% [35]. A solid hypoechoic nodule has an odds ratio of malignancy of 3.8 [52], although up to 55% of thyroid nodules are hypoechoic on ultrasound making this feature in isolation a less specific marker of thyroid malignancy. A taller-than-wide shape is an indirect measure of nodule stiffness caused by the lack of nodule compression under the ultrasound probe [64]. A refractive shadow at the border of a solid lesion [65], marked intra-nodular flow on Doppler (grade III) and decreased elasticity on USE are also noteworthy if present [35].

PTC's occur mostly in solid nodules but may occasionally present as a mixed nodule. When evaluating mixed thyroid nodules on ultrasound, the solid component should be carefully examined for potential features of malignancy such as microcalcifications, an eccentric shape or an acute angle between the solid component and the internal wall of the nodule (Image **12**). Microcalcifications may be more specific for malignancy in mixed nodules compared to other markers of malignancy [66]. Hypervascularity and irregular margins of the solid component are less robust features of malignancy in mixed nodules [28, 67, 68].

Occasionally, extra-thyroidal extension (ETE) may be evident on the ultrasound examination presenting as a bulge or disruption of the thyroid capsule surrounding the nodule [69 - 72] (Images **32-34**). In contrast, capsular abutment (Image **28**) is less specific for ETE and the presence of a continuous capsule with more than 2 mm of normal thyroid tissue around the nodule reduces the risk of microscopic ETE to less than 6%.

The sensitivities, specificities, PPVs and NPVs of each ultrasound feature are illustrated in Table **3**. In essence, no single ultrasound criterion predicts nodule malignancy or benignancy with certainty, especially because some of the commonly cited benign features such as nodule hyperechogenicity or a peripheral halo have also been reported to occur in malignant nodules [63, 73]. While some features such as microcalcifications, hypoechogenicity, taller-than-wide shape and an irregular margin are moderately specific for the detection of thyroid cancer, they have poor sensitivities.

The combination of ultrasound features into patterns of suspicion to characterise the risk of malignancy of thyroid nodules improves the sensitivity and NPV of ultrasound for the detection of thyroid malignancy without compromising on the specificity and allows the recommendation of nodule size cutoffs whereby FNA biopsy may be worthwhile. Inter-observer agreement in thyroid nodule malignancy risk stratification and FNA biopsy recommendation is also enhanced with the use of sonographic patterns [74, 75]. Two commonly used thyroid malignancy risk stratification systems based on sonographic patterns are those of the American Thyroid Association (ATA; Table **4**) and ETA's European Thyroid Imaging Reporting and Data System (EU-TIRADS; Table **5**) [17, 35]. The main difference between the two classification systems is in the description of hypoechoic nodules. The ATA guidelines classify hypoechoic nodules as having an intermediate suspicion for malignancy (10-20%) if no other features of malignancy are present, and as high suspicion for malignancy (70-90%) when associated with other features of malignancy. In contrast, the EU-TIRADS classifies hypoechoic nodules without any other features of malignancy as having an intermediate suspicion for malignancy (6-17%) if the nodule is slightly hypoechoic in relation to surrounding thyroid tissue, and as high suspicion for malignancy (26-87%) when the nodule is markedly hypoechoic compared to the strap muscles, regardless of the presence of other features of malignancy. This explains the much wider range of malignancy risk in the EU-TIRADS high suspicion category compared to that of the ATA.

In contrast to the ATA and ETA guidelines, the American College of Radiology (ACR) TI-RADS [76] advocates a point-based system for the estimation of thyroid nodule malignancy risk and for the determination of nodule size cut-offs for FNA biopsy and follow-up (Table **6**). In a retrospective study of 3422 nodules, the ACR TI-RADS had a higher malignancy yield than the ATA guidelines (14% *vs.* 10%) and benign nodules were less likely to be biopsied (47% *vs.* 78%), although the ACR TI-RADS was less likely than the ATA guidelines to recommend FNA biopsy of malignant nodules (68% *vs.* 76%) [77]. It is essential to point out that the above-described thyroid nodule risk stratification systems are largely geared towards the detection of PTC and have not been evaluated in long-term prospective studies.

It is important to document the change in nodule size or volume at every visit. The ATA guidelines define nodule growth as an increase of 20% or more in 2 or 3 dimensions of the nodule with a minimum increase of 2 mm or more in each dimension, or an increase in nodule volume of 50% or more [35]. An increase in nodule size may be due to underlying malignancy and often warrants further evaluation with FNA, but one must be mindful that up to 90% of benign nodules increase by up to 15% in volume over a 5-year follow-up period [78, 79]. In a retrospective study of 531 benign thyroid nodules [80], one-third of nodules increased in volume by 15-30%, one-third decreased in volume and the remaining one-third of nodules were unchanged during 40-months of follow-up.

In malignant nodules, the size of the nodule at the time of surgery is related to mortality rates and is used for staging the tumour with the American Joint Committee on Cancer tumour, node and metastases (TNM) classification system. Although nodule size does not seem to be associated with the risk of malignancy [26, 81], nodules larger than 4 cm were found in one study to harbour malignancy in 26% of cases and up to 13% of FNA biopsies in this study were false negatives for malignancy [82]. These findings were not confirmed in another study, where nodules larger than 3 cm did not display an increased risk of malignancy or a higher false positive FNA result [83].

Compared to larger thyroid nodules, malignant subcentimetric nodules are less likely to contain microcalcifications and are more likely to be hypoechoic, taller-than-wide and have irregular (spiculated) margins, leading to lower specificity and higher false positive rates of these ultrasound features in subcentimetric nodules [81]. Because subcentimetric thyroid nodules are less likely to represent clinically significant cancers, ultrasound monitoring is usually sufficient although FNA biopsy should be considered in the presence of CLN involvement and possibly in patients with clinical risk factors for thyroid malignancy [35].

Character of Nodules

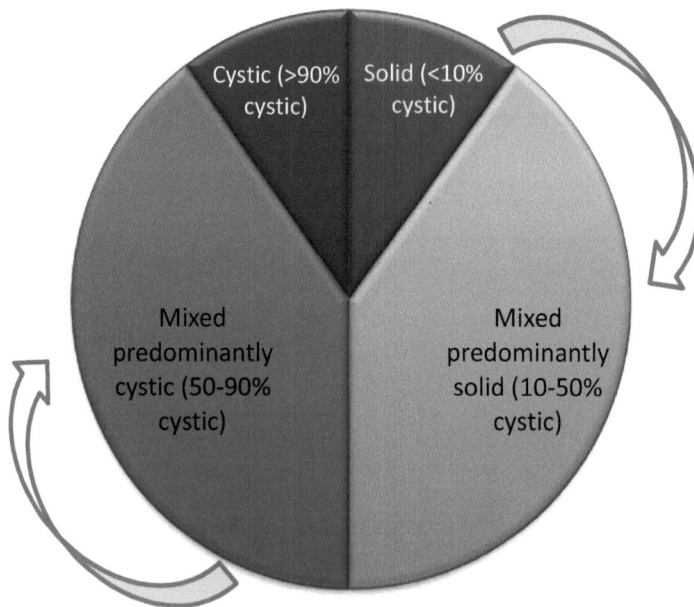

Fig. (5). Character of thyroid nodules based on cystic content.

Table 2. Comparison of ultrasound features of benign and malignant thyroid nodules. Adapted from reference [84] with permission.

Feature	Benign	Malignant
Echogenicity	Isoechoic or hyperechoic	Hypoechoic
Echotexture	Homogeneous	Heterogeneous
Margins	Smooth, well defined, thin peripheral halo	Irregular
AP/transverse dimensions	Wider than tall	Taller than wide
Calcifications	Coarse, complete eggshell or none	Microcalcifications, interrupted eggshell
Vascularity	Peripheral	Central
Spongiform appearance	Yes	No
Lymphadenopathy	No	Yes

Table 3. Ultrasound features of thyroid cancer detailing the sensitivity, specificity, positive predictive value (PPV) and negative predictive value (NPV) of each feature. Adapted from reference [25] with permission.

US Feature	Sensitivity (%)	Specificity (%)	PPV (%)	NPV (%)
Microcalcifications	26.1-59.1	85.8-95.0	24.3-70.7	41.8-94.2
Hypoechogenicity	26.5-87.1	43.4-94.3	11.4-68.4	73.5-93.8
Irregular margins or no halo	17.4-77.5	38.9-85.0	9.3-60.0	38.9-97.8
Solid	69.0-75.0	52.5-55.9	15.6-27.0	88.0-92.1
Central nodular vascularity	54.3-74.2	78.6-80.8	24.0-41.9	85.7-97.4
Taller-than-wide	32.7	92.5	66.7	74.8

Table 4. American Thyroid Association risk stratification of thyroid nodules based on ultrasound characteristics, and recommended nodule size cutoff for FNA biopsy [35] with permission.

Sonographic pattern	Ultrasound features	Estimated risk of malignancy (%)	FNA size cutoff (largest dimension in cm)
High suspicion	Hypoechoic solid nodule or a hypoechoic component of a complex nodule displaying at least one of the following features: ¬ Irregular margins ¬ Microcalcifications ¬ Taller than wide shape ¬ Interrupted rim calcifications with extrusion of soft tissue ¬ CLN involvement	> 70-90	≥ 1

(Table 4) cont.....

Sonographic pattern	Ultrasound features	Estimated risk of malignancy (%)	FNA size cutoff (largest dimension in cm)
Intermediate suspicion	Hypoechoic solid nodule	10-20	≥ 1
Low suspicion	¬ Isoechoic or hyperechoic solid nodule ¬ Complex nodule with an eccentric solid component	5-10	≥ 1.5
Very low suspicion	¬ Complex nodules with a concentric solid component ¬ spongiform nodules	< 3	≥ 2
Benign	Purely cystic nodules	< 1	No biopsy

Table 5. European Thyroid Association risk stratification of thyroid nodules based on ultrasound characteristics, and recommended nodule size cutoff for FNA biopsy. EU-TIRADS: European Thyroid Imaging Reporting and Data System. Adapted from reference [17] with permission.

Category	Ultrasound features	Estimated risk of malignancy (%)	FNA size cutoff (largest dimension in cm)
EU-TIRADS 1: Normal	¬ No nodules on ultrasound	-	No biopsy
EU-TIRADS 2: Benign	¬ Pure cyst ¬ Entirely spongiform	~ 0	No biopsy
EU-TIRADS 3: Low risk	¬ Isoechoic or hyperechoic ovoid nodule with smooth margins	2-4	> 2
EU-TIRADS 4: Intermediate risk	¬ Mildly hypoechoic ovoid nodule with smooth margins	6-17	> 1.5
EU-TIRADS 5: High risk	At least one of the following high suspicion features: ¬ Non-oval shape ¬ Irregular margins ¬ Microcalcifications ¬ Solid nodule with marked hypoechogenicity	26-87	> 1

Table 6. American College of Radiology Thyroid Imaging, Reporting and Data System (TI-RADS) risk stratification of thyroid nodules, and recommended nodule size cut-offs for FNA biopsy and follow-up. TI-RADS: Thyroid Imaging Reporting and Data System. Adapted from reference [76] with permission.

ULTRASOUND FEATURES					
Points	Composition (select 1 feature)	Echogenicity (select 1 feature)	Shape (select 1 feature)	Margins (select 1 feature)	Echogenic Foci (select all that apply)
0	Cystic or spongiform	Anechoic (cystic)	Wider-than-tall	Smooth, Ill-defined or cannot be determined	None or Large (> 1 mm) comet-tail artefacts
1	Mixed	Isoechoic, hyperechoic or cannot be determined	-	-	Macrocalcifications
2	Solid or cannot be determined	Hypoechoic	-	Irregular	Peripheral 'rim' calcifications
3	-	Very hypoechoic	Taller-than-wide	Extra-thyroidal extension	Punctate echogenic foci (with or without comet-tail artefacts)
ADD POINTS					
TI-RADS	Points	Suspicion of malignancy	FNA size cutoff (largest dimension in cm)		Follow-up size cutoff (largest dimension in cm)
1	0	Benign	No biopsy		-
2	2	Not suspicious	No biopsy		-
3	3	Mildly suspicious	≥ 2.5		≥ 1.5
4	4-6	Moderately suspicious	≥ 1.5		≥ 1.0
5	≥ 7	Highly suspicious	≥ 1.0		≥ 0.5

THYROID NODULES – LOW SUSPICION OF MALIGNANCY

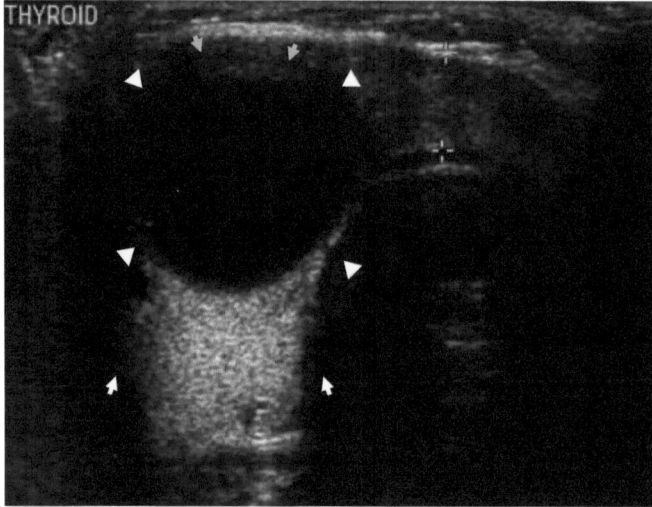

Image (4). Purely cystic right thyroid nodule, transverse plane, with posterior enhancement (white arrows). The nodule is anechoic and the solid-like component at the anterior margin of the cyst is likely due to a reverberation artefact (grey arrows). This nodule has benign features on ultrasound and suspicion of malignancy is less than 1%. FNA biopsy is usually not indicated despite the potentially large size of these nodules.

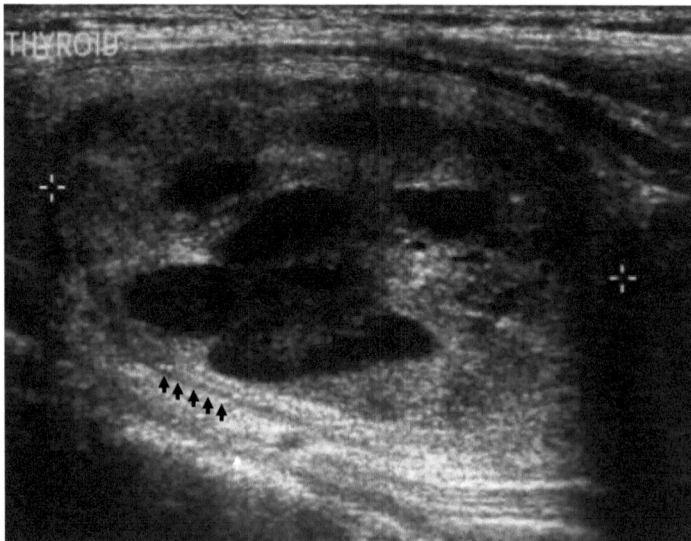

Image (5). Spongiform left thyroid nodule, longitudinal plane, with multiple anechoic cysts that occupy 50% or more of the nodule. Notice the thin peripheral halo (black arrows). Spongiform nodules can be large although suspicion of malignancy is very low (< 3%). FNA biopsy could be considered when clinically indicated in nodules greater than 2 cm in size.

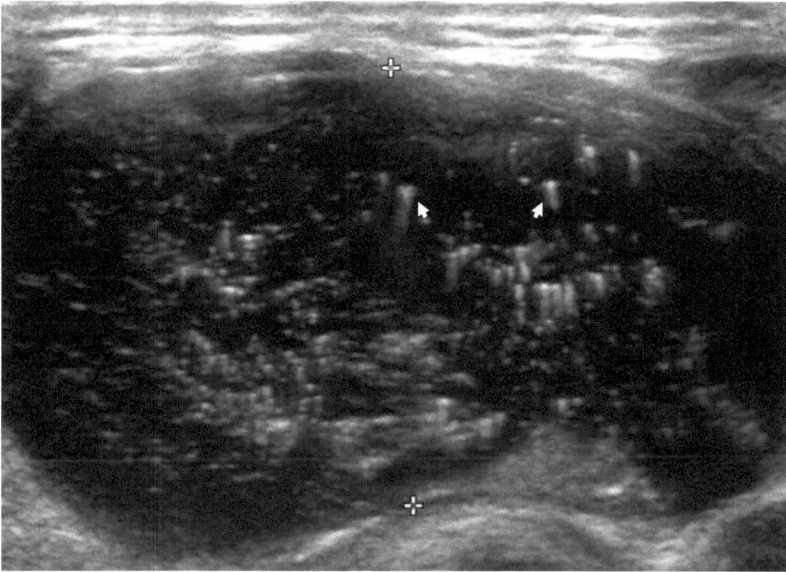

Image (6). Thyroid isthmus colloid cyst displaying innumerable echogenic colloid crystals with a posterior reverberation artefact 'comet tail' (arrows). Suspicion of malignancy is very low (< 3%).

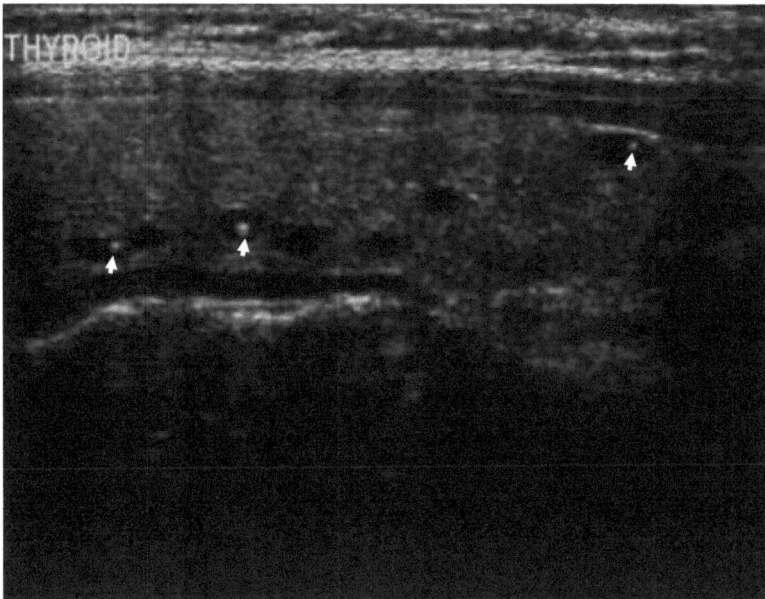

Image (7). Right thyroid lobe, longitudinal plane, displaying multiple small anechoic colloid cysts containing echogenic colloid crystals with the comet tail sign (arrows). Suspicion of malignancy is very low (< 3%).

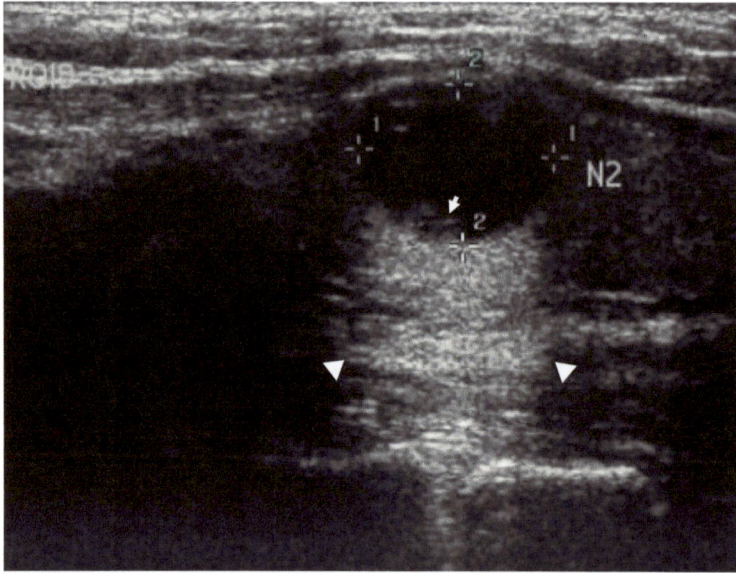

Image (8). Cystic thyroid nodule, longitudinal plane. Note posterior enhancement due to cystic content (arrowheads) and a hyperechoic deposit (arrow) possibly representing debris within the cyst. Suspicion of malignancy is very low (< 3%).

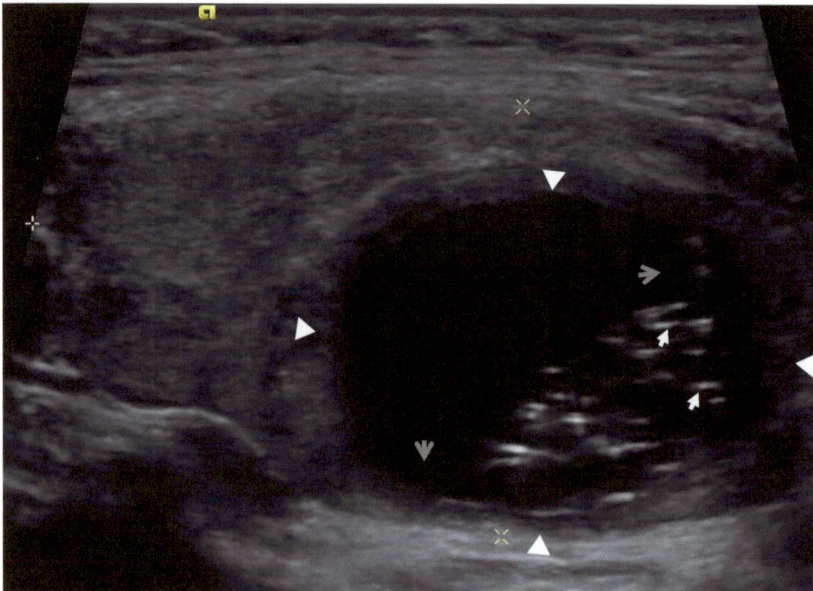

Image (9). Left thyroid mixed nodule, longitudinal plane. The nodule is predominantly cystic and displays a small solid component containing multiple tiny cysts with enhancement of the back walls of the cysts (white arrows). Note the concentric distribution of the solid component with obtuse angles between the solid component and the wall of the nodule (grey arrows). Suspicion of malignancy is very low (< 3%).

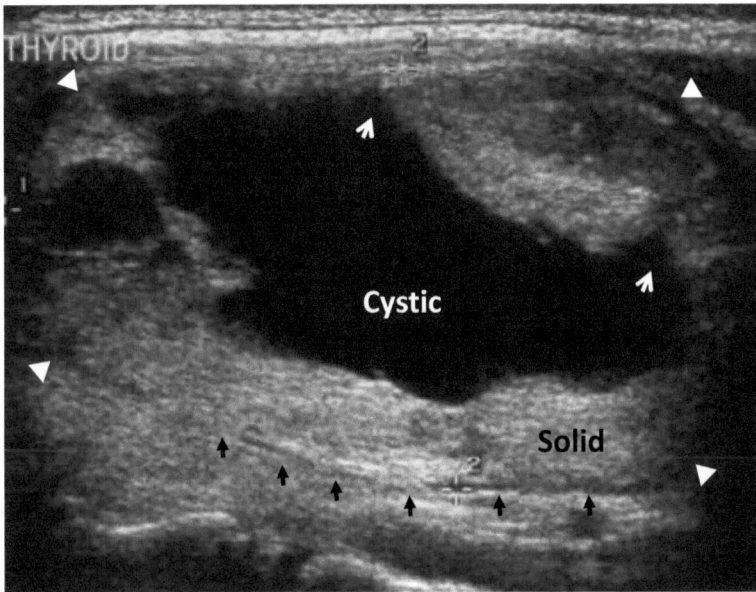

Image (10). Mixed predominantly cystic left thyroid nodule (greater than 50% cystic), longitudinal plane, with a thin peripheral halo (black arrows). Note the concentric distribution of the solid component appearing as a thickening of the nodule wall with obtuse angles between the solid component and the wall of the nodule (white arrows). Suspicion of malignancy is very low (< 3%).

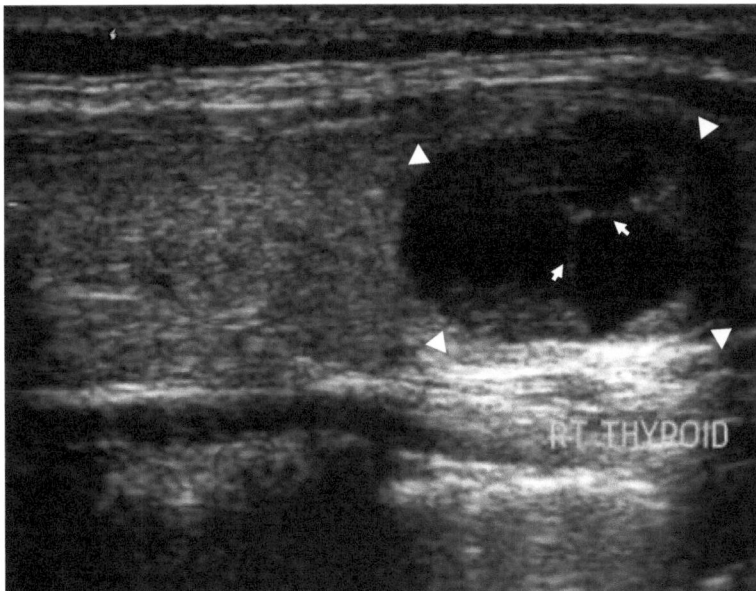

Image (11). Right inferior thyroid nodule, longitudinal plane. The nodule is mixed predominantly cystic with septations (arrows). Note posterior enhancement due to the cystic content of the nodule. Suspicion of malignancy is very low (< 3%).

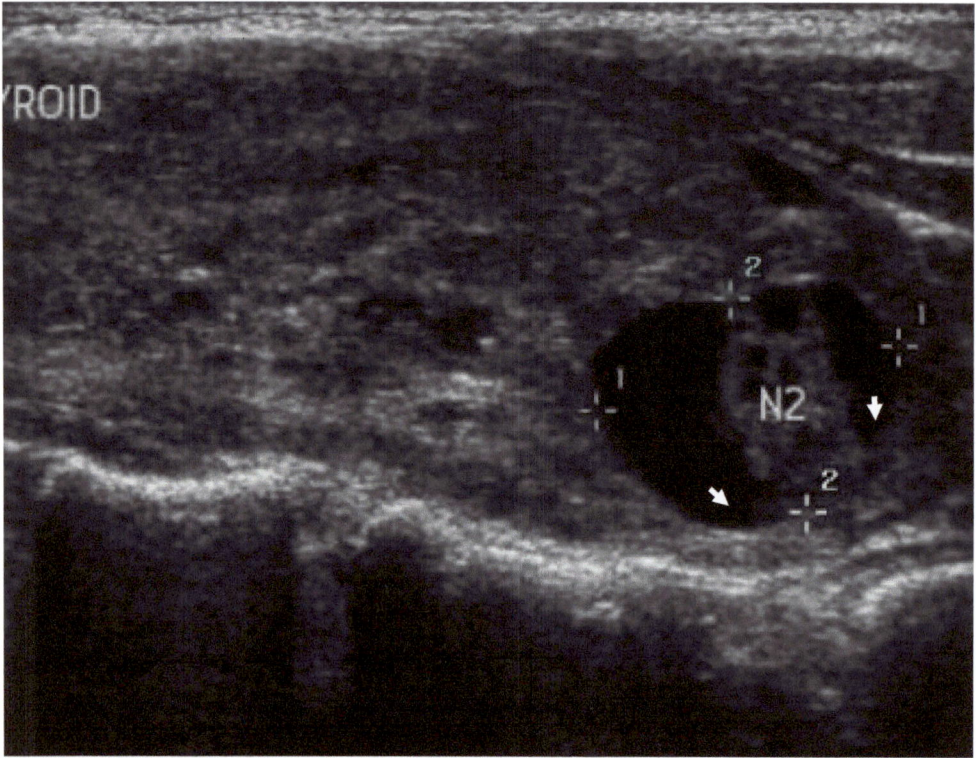

Image (12). Mixed predominantly cystic left inferior thyroid nodule, longitudinal plane, displaying an eccentric solid component with acute angles between the solid component and the wall of the nodule (arrows). Suspicion of malignancy is low (5-10%).

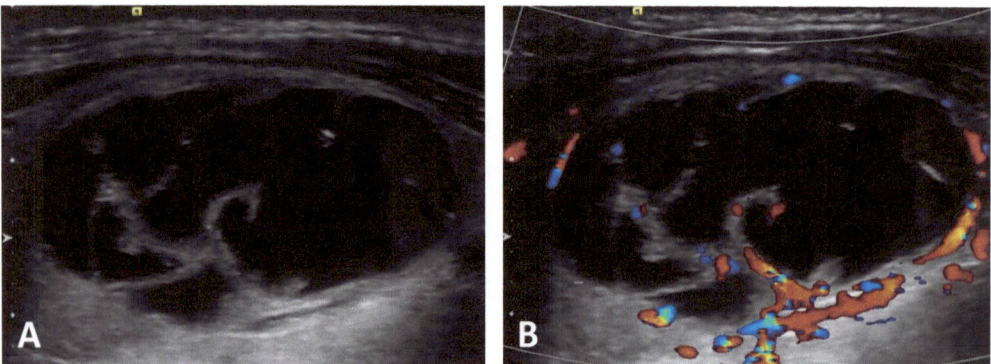

Image (13). Mixed predominantly cystic right thyroid nodule (A), longitudinal plane, displaying papillae-shaped extensions of the solid component and grade II vascularity (B). The presence of an eccentric solid component is associated with an increased suspicion of malignancy on ultrasound, from very low suspicion (< 3%) in the presence of a concentric solid component to low suspicion of malignancy (5-10%)with an eccentric solid component as in this case.

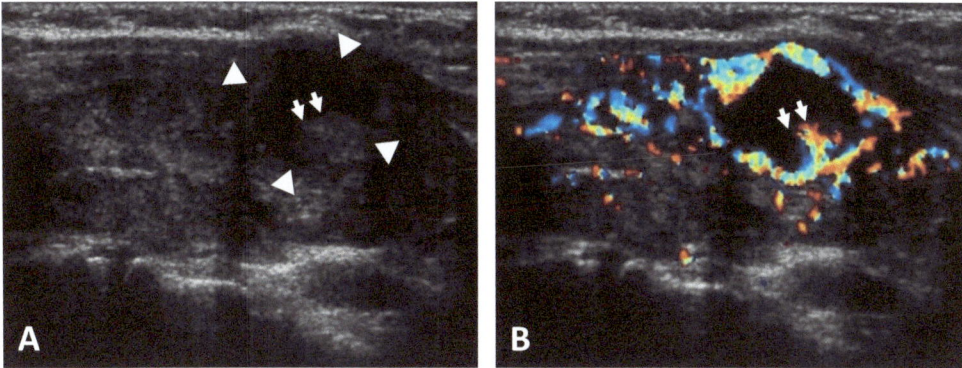

Image (14). Mixed predominantly cystic left thyroid nodule (A), longitudinal plane, displaying peripheral vascularity with high-intensity flow (B) in the small solid component (arrows). The angles between the solid component and the wall of the nodule are obtuse. Suspicion of malignancy is very low (< 3%).

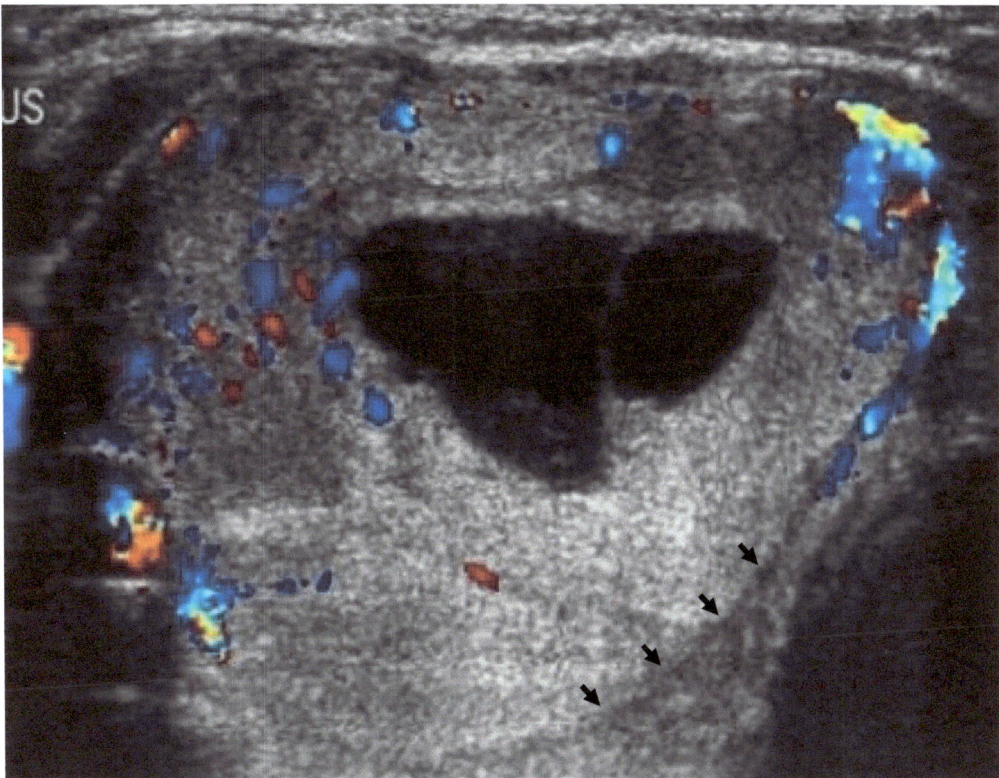

Image (15). Mixed predominantly solid right thyroid nodule, transverse plane, with a septated cystic content occupying 10-50% of the nodule. The nodule exhibits a regular margin with a thin peripheral halo (black arrows) and grade II flow on Doppler. Suspicion of malignancy is low (5-10%).

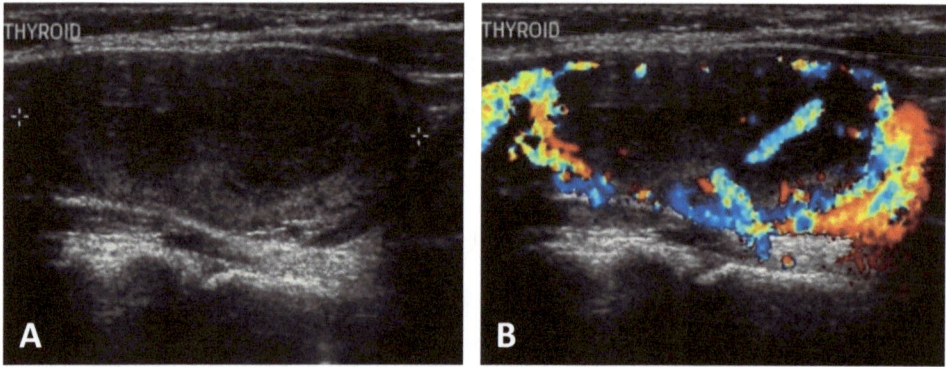

Image (16). Large right thyroid nodule (A), longitudinal plane, demonstrating mostly peripheral flow (grade II vascularity) on Doppler study (B). Suspicion of malignancy: low (5-10%).

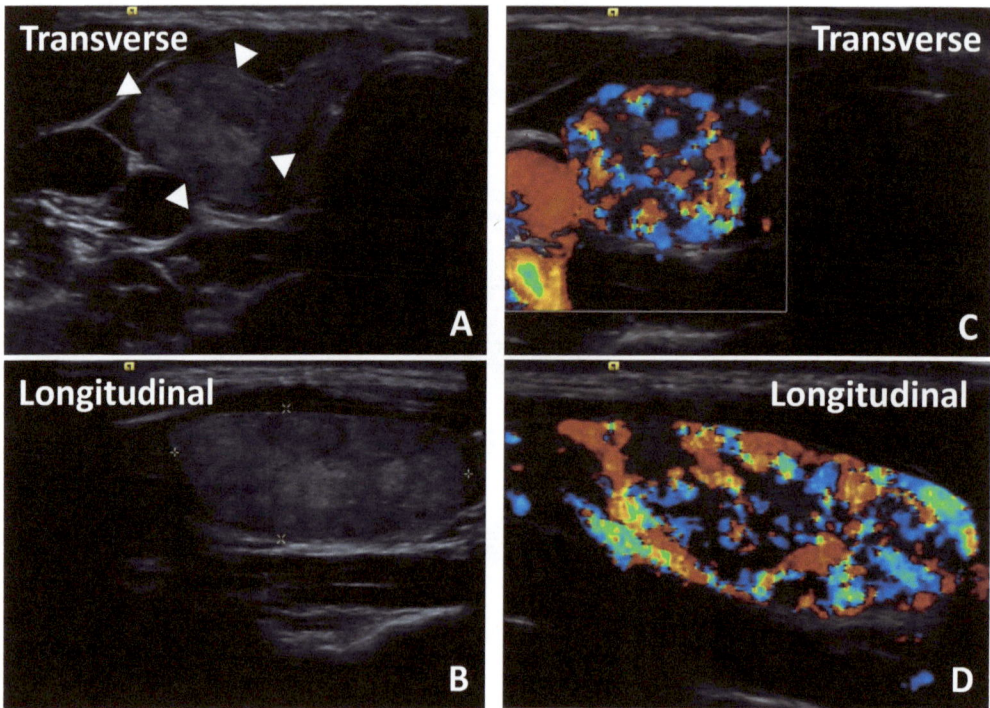

Image (17). Heterogeneous right thyroid nodule, transverse (A) and longitudinal (B) planes, in a patient with Hashimoto's thyroiditis. Note marked intra-nodular flow exceeding 50% of the nodule area (C & D), in addition to peripheral flow on Doppler (grade III vascularity). Suspicion of malignancy: low (5-10%).

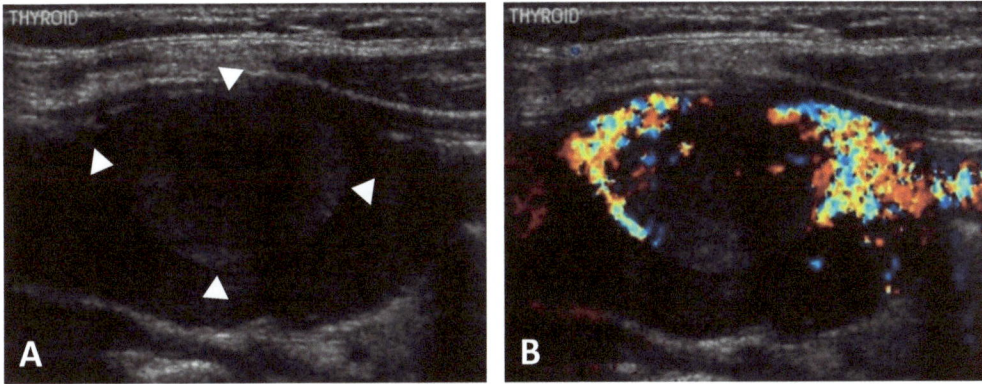

Image (18). Isoechoic left thyroid nodule, longitudinal plane, in a patient with Hashimoto's thyroiditis. Note the smooth well-defined nodule margins, oval shape (A) and peripheral flow on Doppler (B, grade II vascularity). Suspicion of malignancy: low (5-10%).

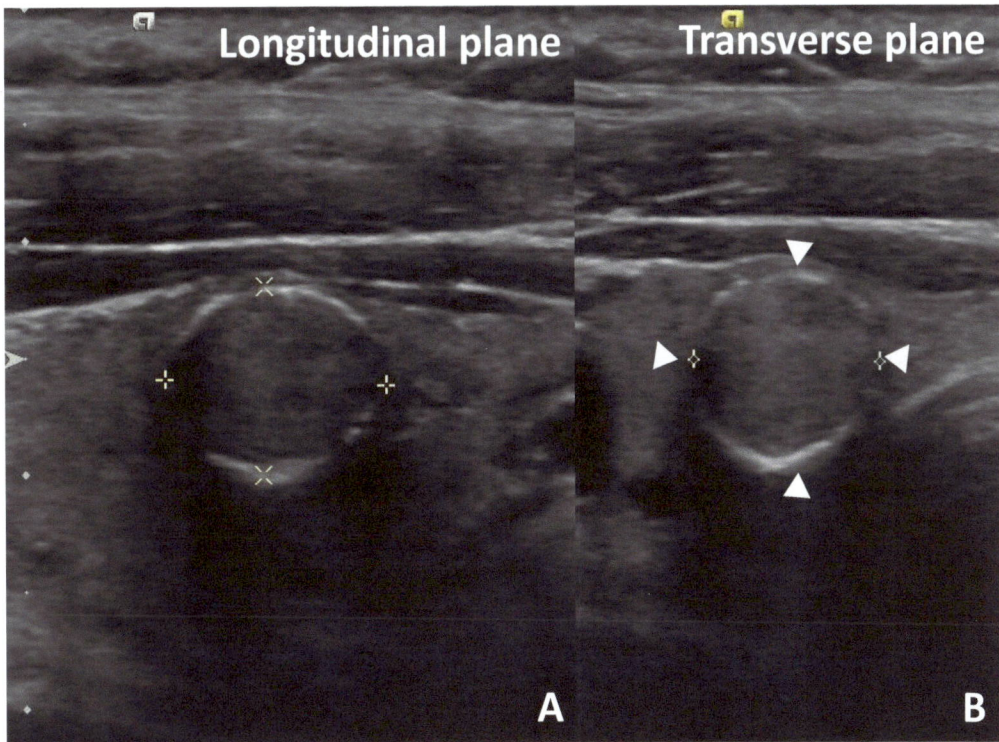

Image (19). Right thyroid nodule displaying rim or 'eggshell' calcification (arrowheads). The nodule is isoechoic and the calcification rim appears intact with no extrusion of thyroid tissue contents beyond the nodule. Suspicion of malignancy: low (5-10%).

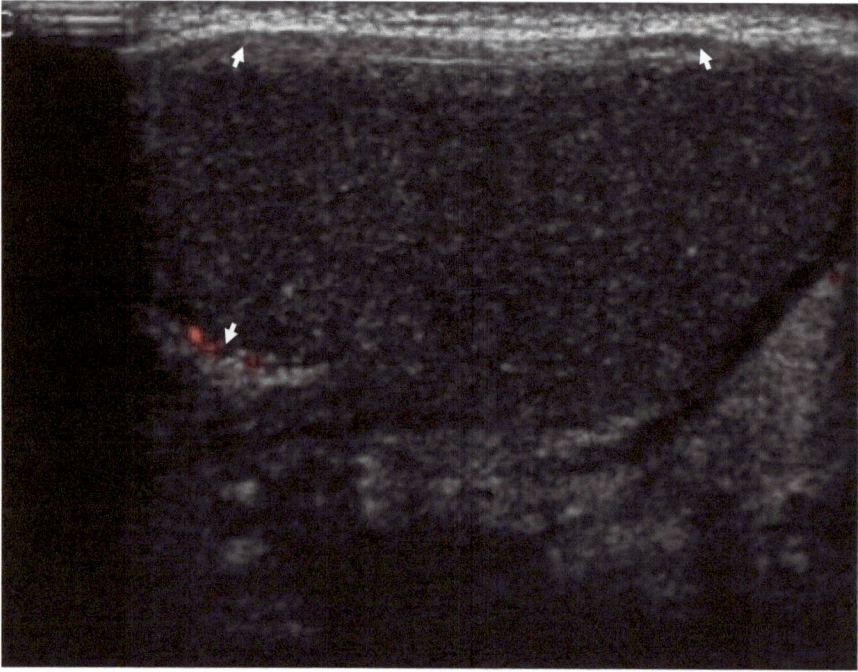

Image (20). Large thyroglossal duct (TGD) cyst located in the midline of the neck superior to the thyroid isthmus. The cyst displays benign features with a suspicion of malignancy less than 1%. Note the thick capsule (arrows), coarse granular echogenicity and absence of Doppler flow inside the cyst. TGD cysts often contain thick proteinaceous material that may be difficult to aspirate. TGD cysts are occasionally involved in thyroid malignancy making their identification and follow-up of clinical importance.

THYROID NODULES: INTERMEDIATE TO HIGH SUSPICION OF MALIGNANCY

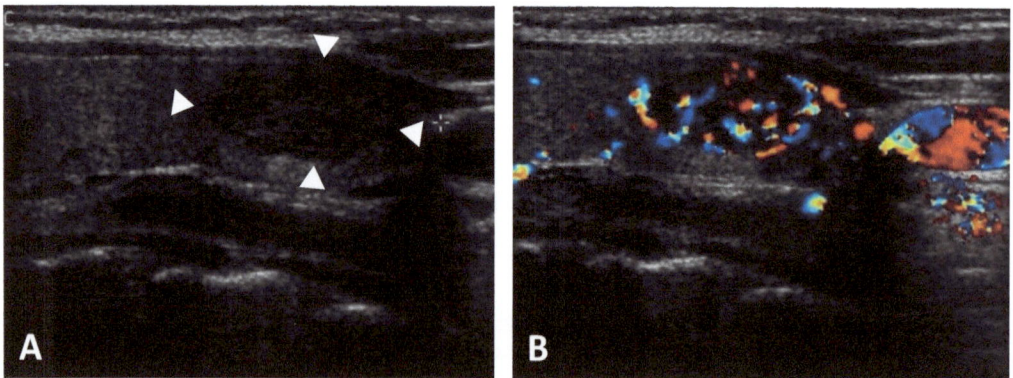

Image (21). Left inferior thyroid nodule, longitudinal plane (A). The nodule is hypoechoic with moderate intensity central flow constituting grade II vascularity (B). Suspicion of malignancy: intermediate (10-20%).

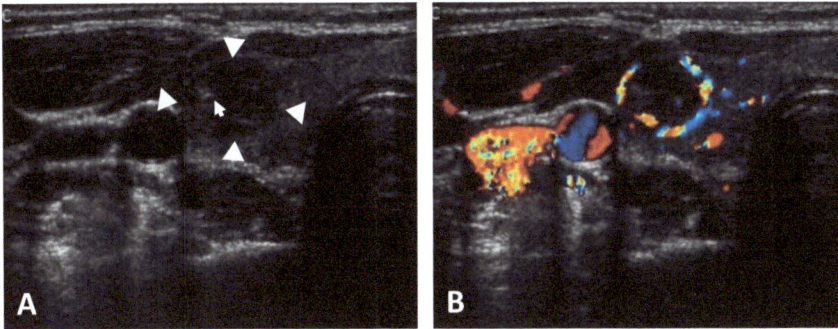

Image (22). Hypoechoic right thyroid nodule, transverse plane (A) with peripheral vascularity (grade II, B). The nodule displays an echogenic focus (arrow) that may represent a colloid deposit, the back wall of a microcyst, or calcification. Such foci are best evaluated in real-time ultrasonography and occasionally an FNA biopsy may be indicated. Suspicion of malignancy: intermediate (10-20%).

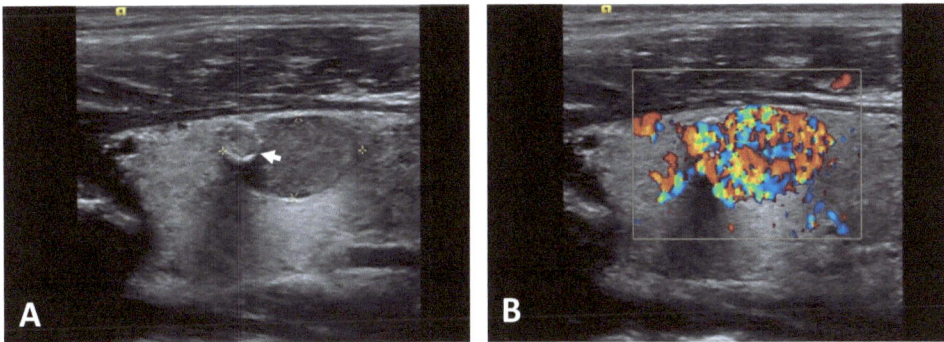

Image (23). Hypoechoic right thyroid nodule, longitudinal plane (A), displaying intense grade III intranodular vascularity on Doppler (B). Note small eggshell calcification (arrow) at the superior corner of the nodule (A). Suspicion of malignancy: intermediate (10-20%).

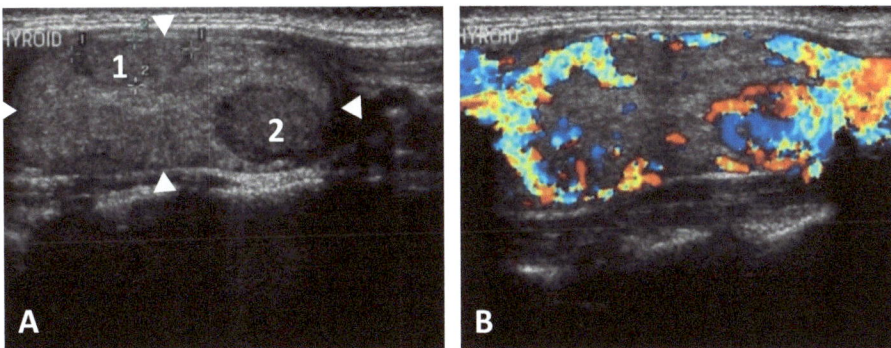

Image (24). Patient with Graves' hyperthyroidism and a heterogeneous right thyroid nodule (arrowheads) in the longitudinal plane (A), demonstrating mostly peripheral flow (grade II vascularity) on Doppler (B). Note two smaller relatively hypoechoic nodules 1 and 2 within the large nodule (A). Nodule 1 displays peripheral vascularity while nodule 2 displays intense intra-nodular flow (B). Suspicion of malignancy: intermediate (10-20%). FNA biopsies of the large nodule and the two smaller nodules were reported benign.

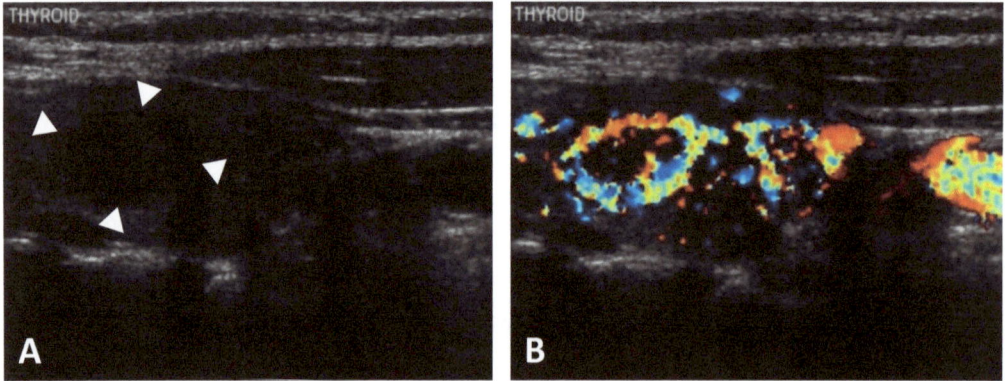

Image (25). Hypoechoic ill-defined right thyroid nodule (A) with grade II vascularity (B), longitudinal plane, in a patient with Hashimoto's thyroiditis. Doppler study helps to delineate the nodule margins. Note the distorted and heterogeneous architecture of the gland with increased vascularity in keeping with chronic thyroiditis.

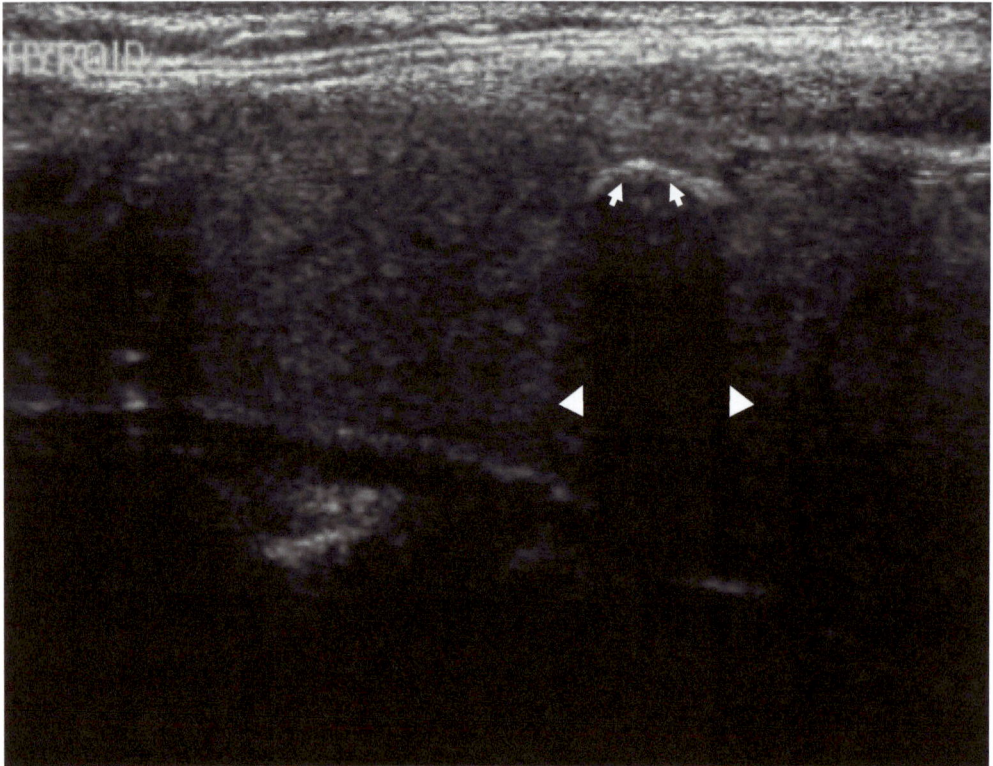

Image (26). Left thyroid nodule, longitudinal plane, displaying partial rim macrocalcification (arrows) with posterior shadowing artefact (arrowheads) which is obscuring the characteristics and posterior border of the nodule.

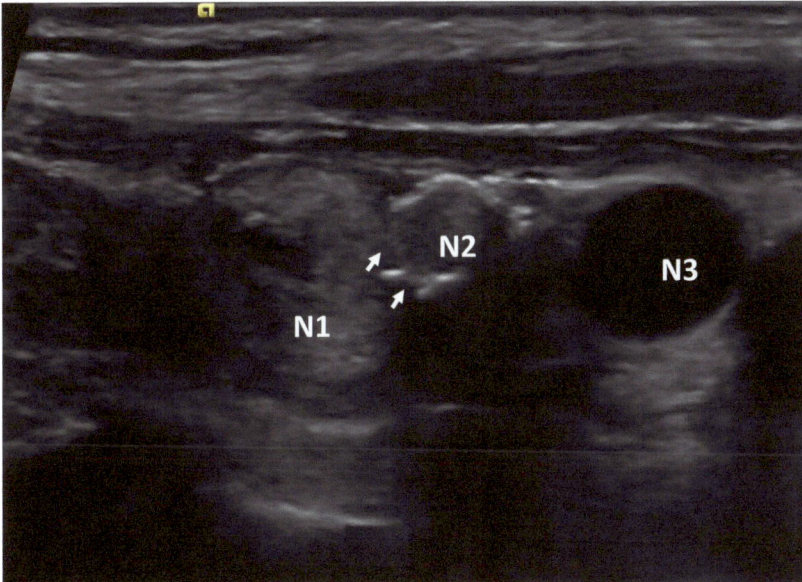

Image (27). Isoechoic right thyroid nodule (N2), longitudinal plane, displaying an interrupted rim calcification (arrows) with no definite soft tissue extrusion on ultrasound. The patient presented with multiple thyroid nodules, nodule N1 is predominantly solid while nodule N3 is purely cystic.

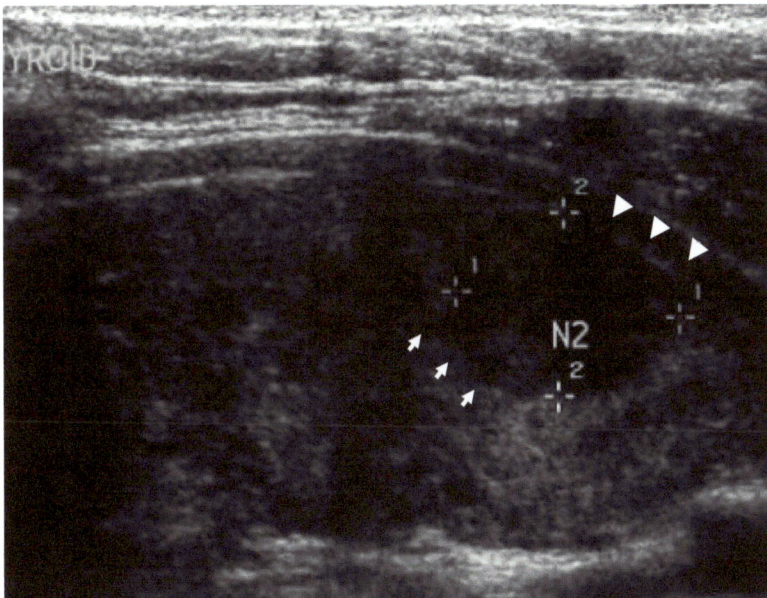

Image (28). Hypoechoic right thyroid nodule, longitudinal plane, with an irregular (infiltrative) posterior margin (arrows). The nodule abuts the thyroid border anteriorly (arrowheads) with no definite extrathyroidal extension. Suspicion of malignancy on ultrasound: high (> 70-90%), FNA biopsy was consistent with papillary thyroid carcinoma.

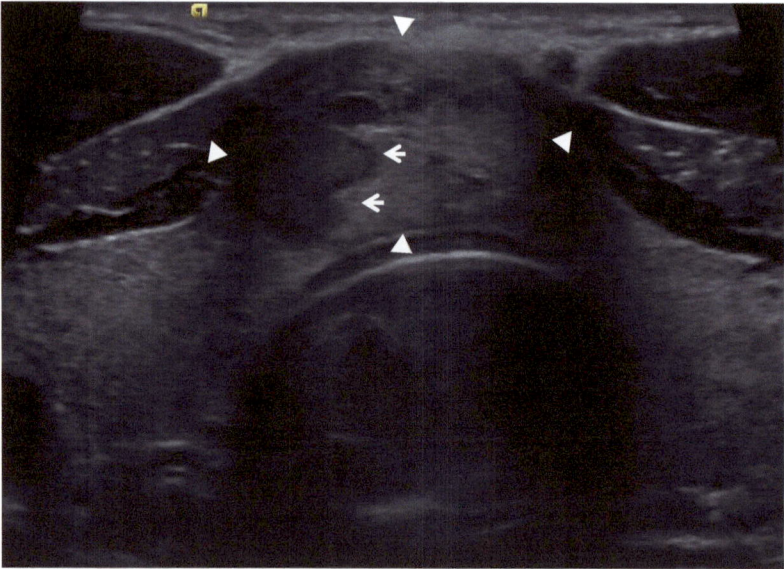

Image (29). Heterogeneous thyroid isthmus nodule (arrowheads). While the nodule is isoechoic, it contains a small hypoechoic focus with irregular lobulated margins (arrows). FNA biopsy of the isoechoic area was reported as benign, whereas the hypoechoic focus proved to be malignant [papillary thyroid carcinoma]. In heterogeneous thyroid nodules, FNA biopsy is best targeted at the more suspicious areas of the nodule to avoid a false negative biopsy result.

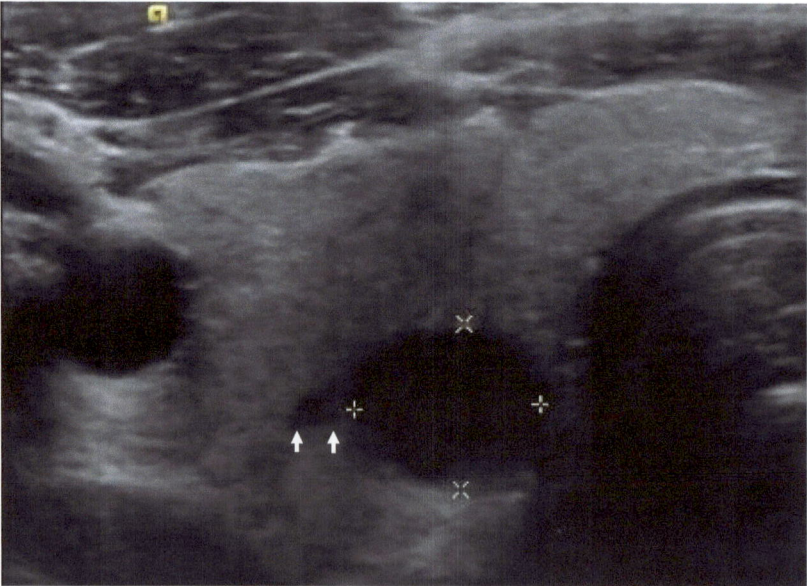

Image (30). Hypoechoic subcentimetric (0.8 cm) right thyroid nodule, transverse plane, displaying a spiculated margin (arrows). FNA biopsy confirmed the diagnosis of papillary thyroid carcinoma.

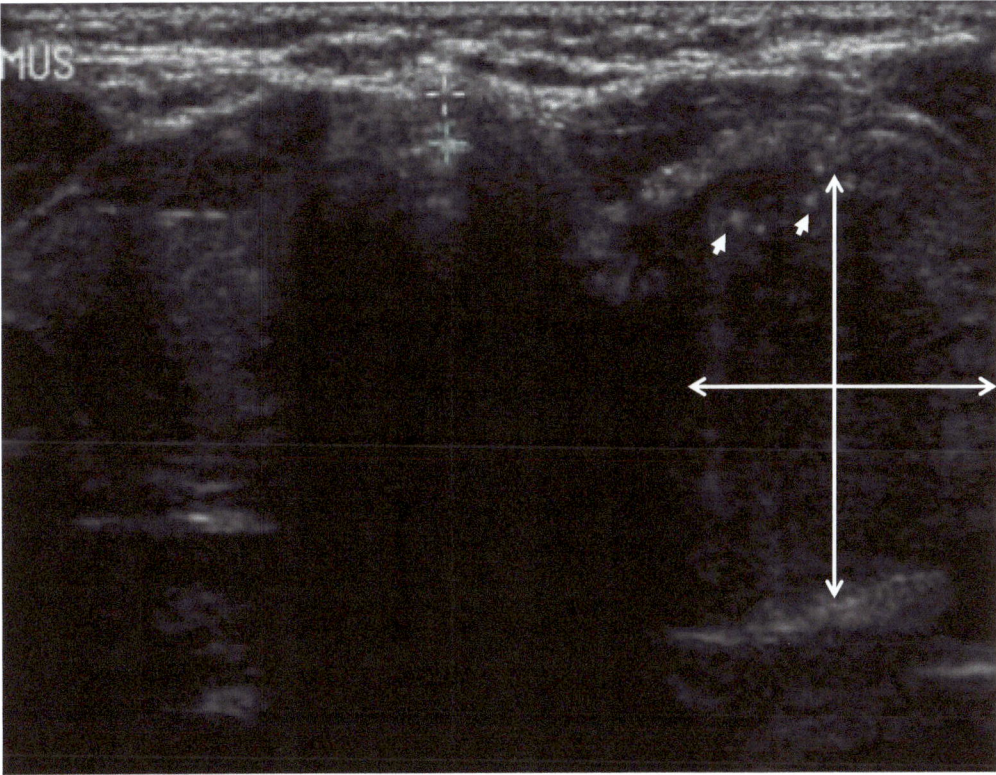

Image (31). Taller-than-wide heterogeneous left thyroid nodule, transverse plane, with microcalcifications (arrows). The anteroposterior-to-transverse diameter ratio was 4:3. FNA biopsy was consistent with papillary thyroid carcinoma.

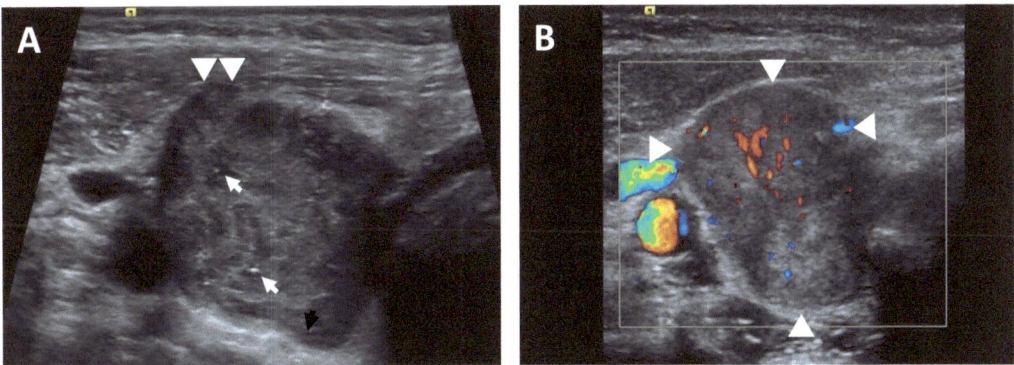

Image (32). Taller-than-wide hypoechoic right thyroid nodule, transverse plane (A), displaying irregular margins (black arrow), microcalcifications (white arrows), and extrathyroidal-extension beyond the thyroid border anteriorly (arrowheads). Note minimal intra-nodular vascularity (B). Histopathology report was consistent with papillary thyroid carcinoma, tall-cell variant.

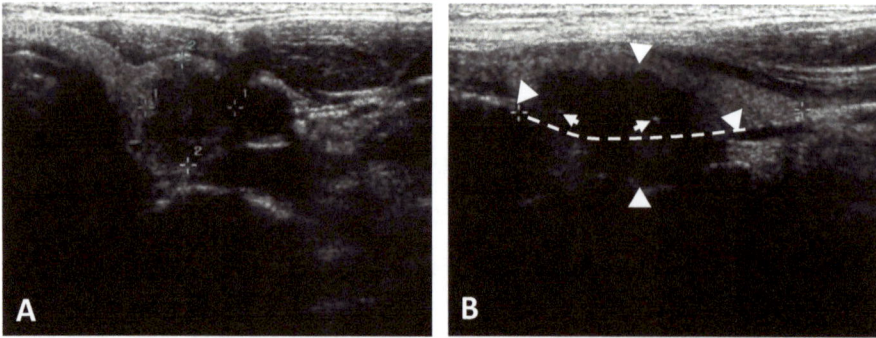

Image (33). Hypoechoic left thyroid nodule, transverse (A) and longitudinal (B) planes, displaying infiltrative irregular margins, microcalcifications (arrows, B) and a high suspicion of malignancy. Extrathyroidal extension is evident at the posterior margin of the thyroid border (dotted line, B). FNA biopsy was reported as papillary thyroid carcinoma.

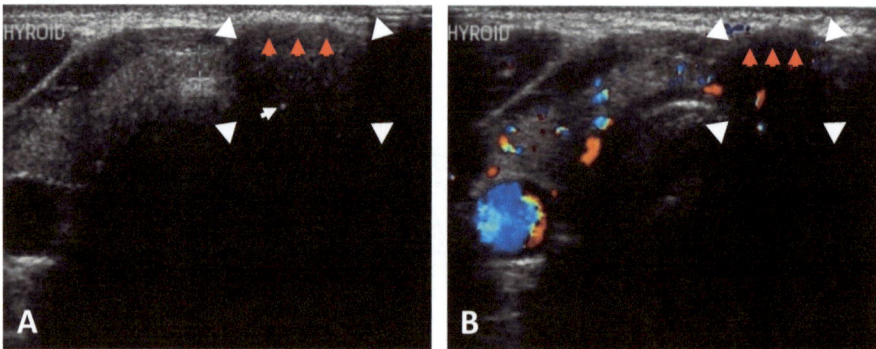

Image (34). Hypoechoic left isthmus nodule, transverse plane (A), displaying grade I vascularity (B), micro-calcifications (white arrow, A), ill-defined margins and extension beyond the anterior border of the thyroid gland (red arrows). Suspicion of malignancy: high (> 70-90%). FNA biopsy was reported as medullary thyroid carcinoma.

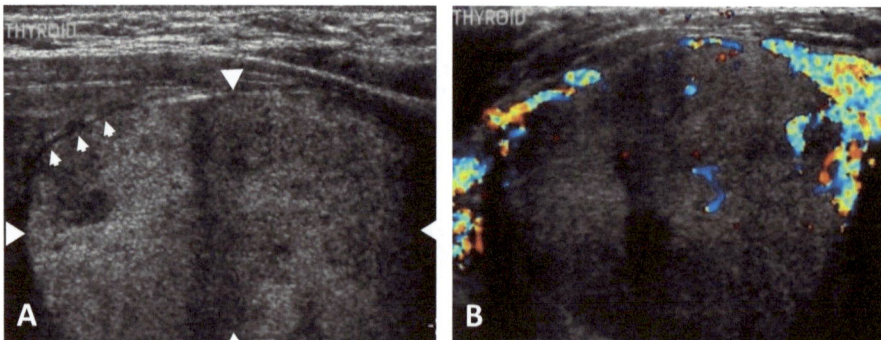

Image (35). Large, taller-than-wide, isoechoic left thyroid nodule, longitudinal (A) and transverse (B) planes, with grade II peripheral vascularity (B). The post-operative pathology report was consistent with the follicular variant of papillary thyroid carcinoma. In contrast to classical PTC, note the well-defined regular margins (arrowheads), peripheral hypoechoic halo (arrows) and absence of calcifications (A). Follicular thyroid cancer has similar ultrasound features to the follicular variant of papillary thyroid carcinoma.

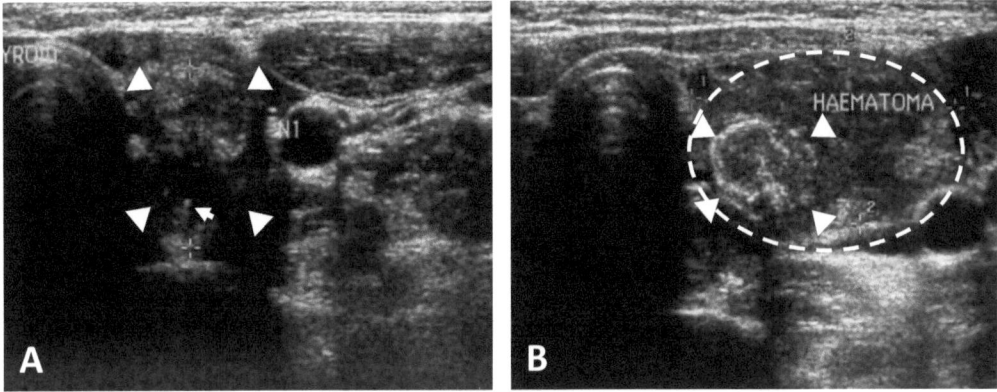

Image (36). Left thyroid gland, transverse plane (A), displaying an ill-defined heterogeneous nodule, taller-than-wide with microcalcifications (arrow). Suspicion of malignancy: high (> 70-90%). FNA biopsy was reported as papillary thyroid carcinoma. The dotted circle outlines the extent of a post-FNA biopsy haematoma (B) with enhancement of the nodule margins (white arrowheads).

CHAPTER 5

Ultrasound of Cervical Lymph Nodes

Abstract: Ultrasound examination of the anterior cervical lymph nodes constitutes an important component of thyroid ultrasound. Up to 30% of thyroid cancer patients are found to have cervical lymph node metastasis on the pre-operative ultrasound examination, leading to altered surgical management. There are six anterior cervical lymph node compartments that are examined systematically on ultrasound beginning with compartments I and VI/VII, followed by compartments II, III and IV and finally compartment V. Low-suspicion cervical nodes are oval in shape with an intact fatty hilum and central vascularity. Intermediate suspicion nodes are those with an absent hilum and round shape defined as a nodal long-axis to short-axis ratio less than 2, or a short-axis ≥ 8 mm in compartment II nodes and ≥ 5 mm in compartments III and IV and VI. In addition to these changes, high suspicion nodes display one or more of the following features: microcalcifications, cystic change, hyperechoic component, irregular margins, and/or peripheral/chaotic vascularity. Nodal microcalcifications and cystic changes on ultrasound have the highest specificity for metastatic thyroid cancer followed by hyperechogenicity, peripheral vascularity and a round shape. Suspicious cervical nodes should be further evaluated with ultrasound-guided fine needle aspiration biopsies and measurement of tumour markers in the needle washout.

Keywords: Cervical lymph node, Cystic content, Fatty hilum, Fine needle aspiration, Long-axis, Metastasis, Microcalcifications, Peripheral vascularity, Power Doppler, Short-axis, Steinkamp's ratio, Thyroid cancer, Trachea-oesophageal groove, Tumour markers, Ultrasound.

Evaluation of the central and lateral CLN compartments is an essential part of neck ultrasonography. There are more than 300 CLN in the neck and it is common to see CLNs in the majority of patients, including those who had total thyroidectomy for thyroid cancer. The size, number and ultrasound characteristics of CLNs may vary with age whereby younger patients less than 40 years of age tend to have a greater number of nodes, whereas the nodes are larger with a greater incidence of a well-defined echogenic hilum in older patients [85].

Ultrasound scanning of CLNs is undertaken with a linear transducer at frequency 12 MHz for superficial nodes and 8-10 MHz for deeper nodes. Power Doppler is preferable to colour Doppler for the detection of central hilar vascularity and any

Samer El-Kaissi & Jack R Wall

abnormal vascularization of the node. The patient should be supine with the neck extended comfortably in the same position as that for the thyroid ultrasound examination. This allows imaging of nodes in the lower part of compartments IV and VI. Imaging is undertaken in the transverse plane initially and any abnormalities are investigated further in the longitudinal plane and using Doppler flow. All CLN compartments are assessed in a systematic fashion starting with compartments I and VI, followed by compartments II, III and IV and finally compartment V. Towards the end of the examination, the transducer is angled inferiorly in order to image compartment VII nodes. It may also be helpful to have the patient turn their head to the side in order not to miss nodes in the trachea-oesophageal groove [86].

A pre-operative neck ultrasound in patients with thyroid cancer is critical for identifying any suspicious CLNs, allows ultrasound-guided FNA (UG-FNA) and measurement of biochemical tumour markers in the needle washout. In patients with PTC, the detection of metastatic CLN often alters the initial surgical approach, prevents the need for re-operation, and may improve the overall and disease-free survival [87].

CLN metastases are seen in 20-30% of thyroid cancer patients on the pre-operative neck ultrasound [88, 89] with the central compartment as the most commonly involved site [90]. Approximately half of the malignant CLNs are present in compartments III and IV, and the other half in compartment VI [91]. Thyroid cancer usually metastasises to the ipsilateral cervical lymph nodes, but the contralateral CLNs are affected in up to 20% of cases [88, 92]. The presence of CLN metastases in the absence of a malignant thyroid nodule may suggest the presence of an unusually aggressive thyroid microcarcinoma [93] (Image **41**).

Ultrasound appears to be as accurate as other imaging modalities for the detection of CLN metastases before surgery [94] but lacks sensitivity for the detection of malignant central CLNs in patients with intact thyroid glands. Pre-operative cross-sectional imaging of the neck with CT or MRI is usually reserved for patients with suspected invasive thyroid cancer to assess the extent of ETE. In one retrospective analysis, more than 70% of PTC patients and no evidence of central CLN on the pre-operative ultrasound were found to have central CLN metastasis at the time of surgery, but the clinical significance of this phenomenon is unknown as there was no difference in disease-free and recurrence-free survival of patients with central node metastasis compared to those without node metastasis [95]. Similar studies have cast doubt on the benefits of prophylactic central CLN dissection in patients undergoing total thyroidectomy for DTC.

On ultrasound, CLNs can be classified as having a low, intermediate or a high suspicion for malignancy (Table **7**) [86]. Low suspicion CLNs (Image **37**) appear oval-shaped with a hypoechoic periphery and an echogenic vascular 'fatty' hilum in the centre. While the presence of a normal hilum reduces suspicion of malignancy, visualization of the hilum on ultrasound is highly variable, ranging from 28-87% in different studies [91, 96, 97], and is possibly influenced by the location of the nodes and skill of the sonographer. Therefore, the inability to visualize a fatty hilum in CLNs without any other suspicious features should not be interpreted as abnormal. Hilar vascularity is seen in approximately two-thirds of normal CLNs, occasionally without an apparent hilum on grey-scale examination. On the other hand, peripheral vascularity has been reported to occur in up to 18% of benign CLNs [91, 96, 97].

CLNs affected by malignancy often display similar ultrasound features to those seen in the malignant thyroid nodule and while no single ultrasonographic feature is diagnostic of malignancy, the following features increase the suspicion of nodal metastases [98]:

1. Loss of hilar architecture and/or nodal hyperechogenicity (Image **43**).
2. Round shape (Images **38** and **43**) – short-axis (SA) diameter greater than 8 mm in level II nodes or greater than 5 mm in level III, IV and VI nodes [86]. A long-axis (LA) to SA ratio less than 2, known as Steinkamp's ratio, may be a more accurate measure of the round shape of a node than the SA alone and is associated with an increased risk of nodal malignancy [99]. It is noteworthy that up to 36% of benign nodes are non-ovoid with a LA/SA ratio < 2 [91, 96, 97, 100]. In the authors' experience, non-ovoid CLNs are commonly seen in compartments I and II, and in patients with Hashimoto's thyroiditis in compartment VI.
3. Microcalcifications (Images **39** and **43**) are typically seen in metastatic PTC but may also occur with MTC.
4. Cystic changes – suggestive of metastatic PTC (Images **41** and **43**)
5. Peripheral vascularity on colour flow Doppler (Images **40** and **43**) – this feature may be easier to appreciate with power Doppler. In contrast, the presence of hilar vascularization is a sign of benignancy.
6. Irregular or ill-defined margins (Images **42** and **43**) due to extension of the malignancy to the capsule of the node. This feature is often associated with increased nodal size.

Less well-characterized potential features of nodal metastases include [98]:

1. Large nodal size – CLNs exceeding 4 cm in their greatest dimension often demonstrate other features of malignancy such as an irregular nodal margin, although increased node size in the absence of other sonographic features of

malignancy is not concerning.

2. Multiple or matted nodes in one or more compartments may occur in malignancy. This is also a common feature of lymphoma and inflammatory conditions such as tuberculosis.

3. Increased nodal stiffness on USE, while not widely used, seems promising with one study suggesting 100% specificity for the detection of nodal malignancy [101]. In this study, the sensitivity of USE was 83% and improved to 92% when combined with grey-scale features.

Importantly, the CLN shape and architecture are more relevant than nodal size in assessing the risk of malignancy as shown in Table 7 [86]. Despite their low-intermediate sensitivity for thyroid cancer metastasis, nodal microcalcifications and cystic changes on ultrasound have the highest specificity for metastatic DTC followed by hyperechogenicity, peripheral vascularity and round shape as shown in Table 8 [86] .

If a positive finding would change management, suspicious nodes greater than 8-10 mm in their smallest diameter, usually their SA dimension, can be further evaluated with UG-FNA [35].

Table 7. Risk stratification of cervical lymph nodes based on ultrasound characteristics. CLN can be stratified on ultrasound as low, intermediate or high suspicion for malignancy. LA – long axis, SA – short axis. Adapted from reference [86] with permission.

Low suspicion	Intermediate suspicion	High suspicion (at least one feature)

Preserved hilum
Normal size
Ovoid shape
Normal or absent hilar vascularity
No suspicious features
	Absent fatty hilum and round shape as defined by:
	- LA/SA ratio < 2
	and/or
	- Increased SA
	  - ≥ 8 mm in compartment II
	  - > 5 mm in compartments III and IV and VI
		Microcalcifications
		Cystic content
		Peripheral or diffuse vascularization
		Hyperechoic (thyroid-like) tissue

Table 8. Reported sensitivities and specificities of ultrasound features of malignant cervical lymph nodes. Adapted from reference [86] with permission.

Sign	Sensitivity (%)	Specificity (%)
Microcalcifications	5-69	93-100
Cystic aspect	10-34	91-100
Peripheral vascularity	40-86	57-93
Hyperechogenicity	30-87	43-95
Round shape	37	70

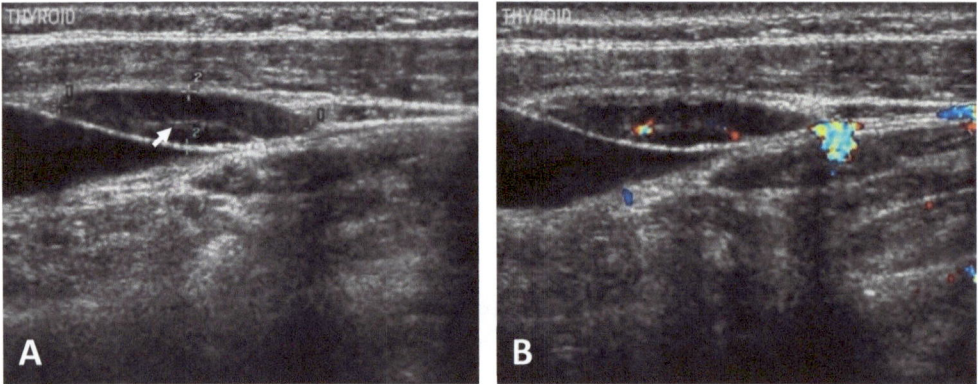

Image (37). Ovoid lateral neck cervical lymph node, long axis. The lymph node is hypoechoic with regular margins and a preserved fatty hilum (arrow, A). Vascularity is normal on Doppler study (B). These features are suggestive of a benign lymph node.

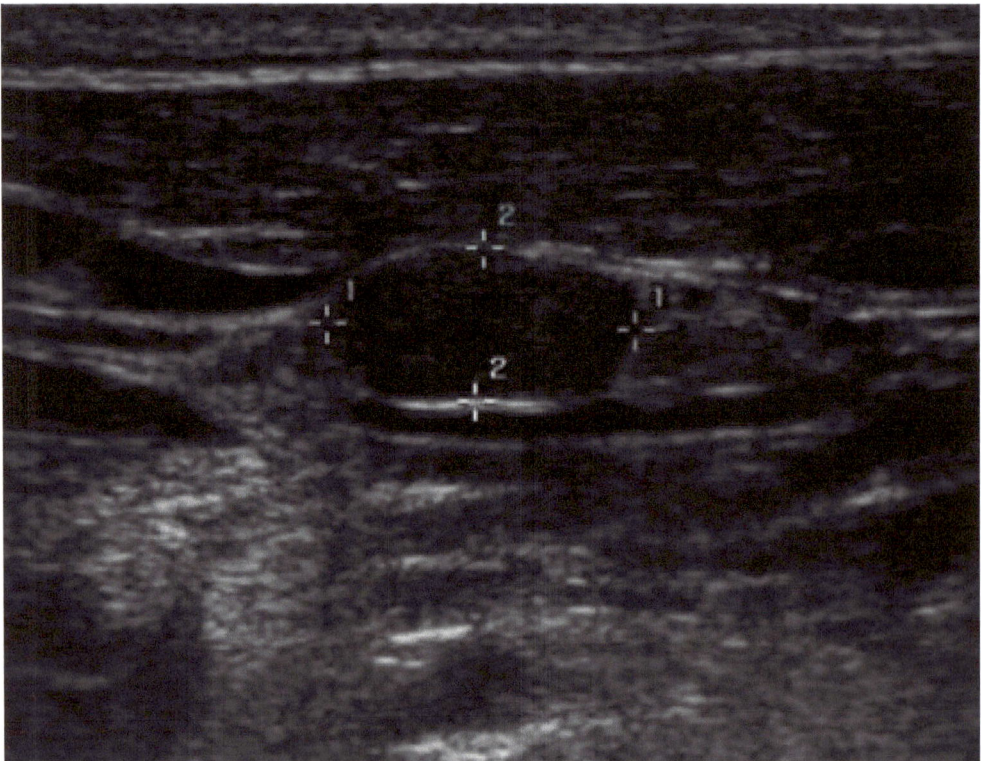

Image (38). Left lateral neck cervical lymph node, long-axis, in a patient with medullary thyroid carcinoma. The node is round (long axis-short axis ratio 1.6) with loss of fatty hilum. Suspicion of malignancy: intermediate.

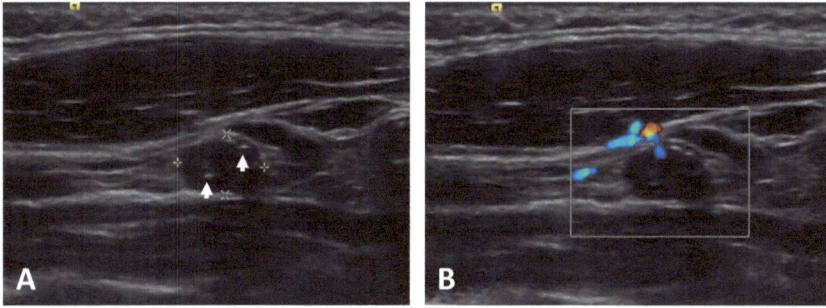

Image (39). Left neck central compartment lymph node (A) displaying a round shape (long axis-short axis ratio 1.6), calcifications (arrows) and an absent fatty hilum. The patient has a history of papillary thyroid carcinoma with cervical lymph node metastases, status post-total thyroidectomy. There was no significant intra-nodal flow on Doppler (B) and while the absence of hilar vascularity may be a normal finding, the presence of calcifications is highly suspicious for recurrent papillary thyroid carcinoma.

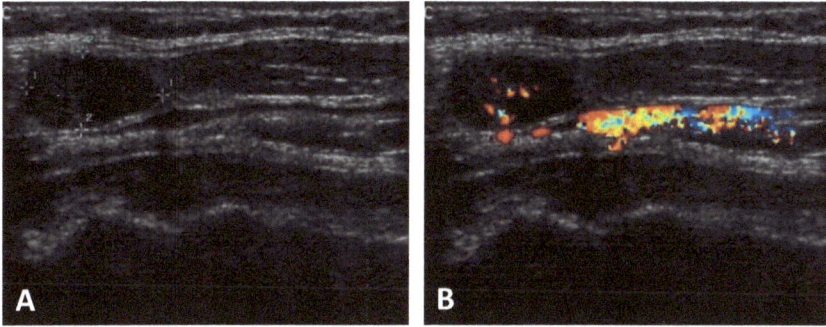

Image (40). Right compartment III cervical lymph node, long-axis, in a patient with a history of differentiated thyroid carcinoma. Note absence of the central hilum (A), round shape suggested by long axis-short axis ratio of 1.5, and chaotic flow pattern on Doppler (B). Suspicion of malignancy: high.

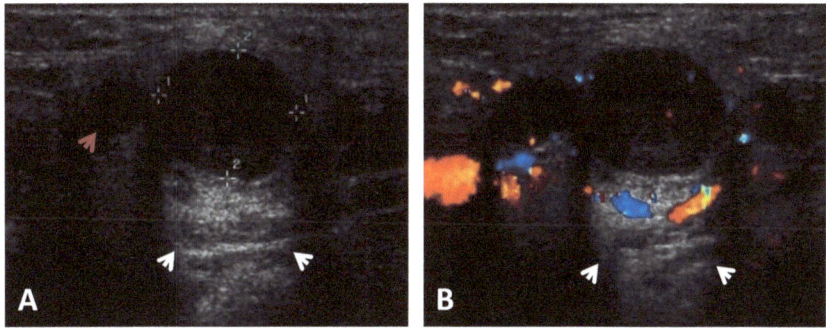

Image (41). Right IB cervical lymph node (A) in a patient with a cytologically benign subcentimetric thyroid nodule. The node is round without a visible fatty hilum and displays cystic content as evidenced by the posterior enhancement (white arrows). A smaller adjacent node is also seen (red arrow, A). Doppler study (B) is often non-contributory in cystic nodes. While the round shape and absence of a central hilum are not uncommon for nodes in compartments I, II and VI, the presence of cystic content as suggested by posterior enhancement is pathognomonic. Suspicion of malignancy: high.

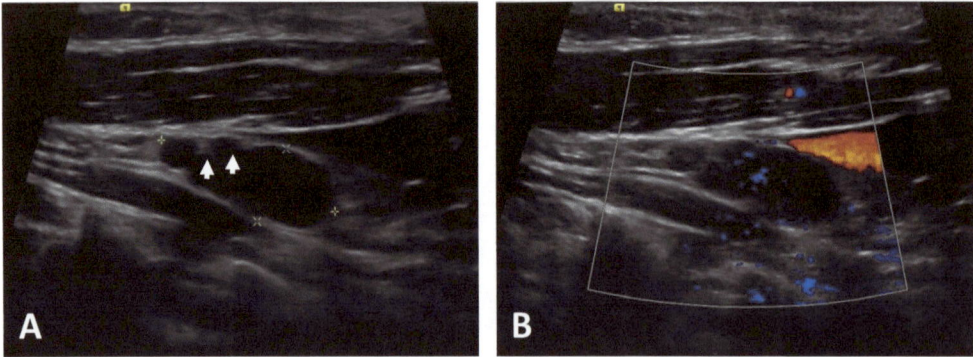

Image (42). Right neck central lymph node with an absent fatty hilum (A) and irregular margins (arrows). The patient has a history of papillary thyroid carcinoma with cervical lymph node metastases, status post-total thyroidectomy. Despite retaining its oval shape and no evidence of abnormal vascularity on Doppler (B), the irregular margins make the node highly suspicious for recurrent papillary thyroid carcinoma.

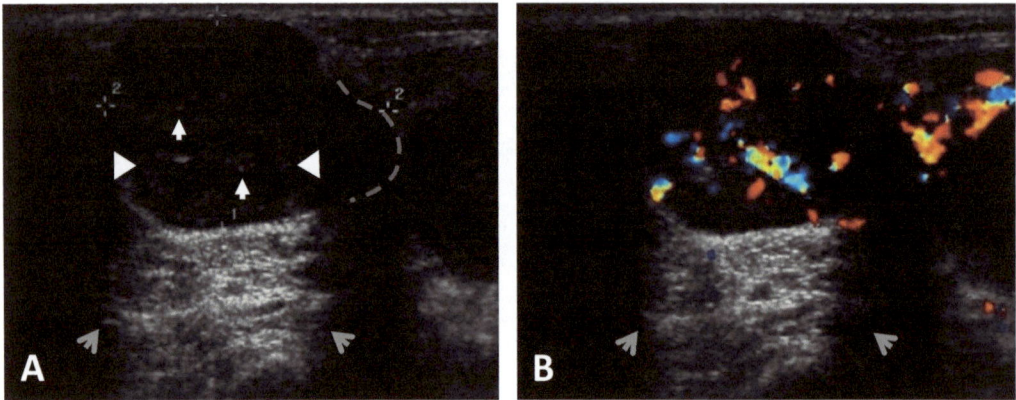

Image (43). Pathological right lateral cervical lymph node. The node is heterogeneous with loss of fatty hilum, round shape, heterogeneous tissue-like material (arrowheads, A) displaying microcalcifications (arrows, A), with an irregular nodal margin (dotted line, A), non-central chaotic Doppler flow (B), and is partially cystic with posterior enhancement (grey arrows). Suspicion of malignancy: high.

CHAPTER 6

Ultrasound-Guided Fine Needle Aspiration Biopsy

Abstract: UG-FNA biopsy of the thyroid and CLNs is a safe and inexpensive procedure that can be performed in the office. Complications such as hematoma and severe pain are uncommon and the procedure provides a greater yield and is more accurate than FNA by palpation. A baseline thyroid ultrasound is essential for determining which nodules and/or CLNs require FNA biopsy and for selecting an entry path. The needle path is either parallel or perpendicular to the ultrasound beam, where the parallel path requires more practice but may be safer as it allows visualization of the biopsy needle throughout the procedure. Negative pressure 'aspiration' or capillary action biopsies are equally effective and a 25-27G needle is usually sufficient for solid nodules, whereas a larger gauge needle may be required for the aspiration of cystic content. The risk of a hematoma post-FNA biopsy is very low although it is important to minimize the number of FNA passes, apply gentle compression at the biopsy site after each pass, and to perform a brief ultrasound scan of the biopsy site at the end of the procedure. It is unclear if holding anti-thrombotic agents before the procedure is beneficial but it is important to ensure that in patients taking warfarin the international normalized ratio (INR) is less than 2.5-3.0 before the procedure. In addition to cytopathology, FNA biopsy allows measurement of tumour markers such as thyroglobulin and calcitonin when clinically indicated. The Bethesda system and the UK Royal College of Pathologists grading system are commonly used for reporting thyroid cytopathology.

Keywords: Anti-thrombotic agent, Bethesda, Biopsy, Benign, Capillary FNA, Calcitonin, Cytopathology, Fine needle aspiration, Hematoma, Lymph node, Malignant, Parathyroid, Thyroid, Thyroglobulin, Ultrasound.

The widespread use of thyroid FNA biopsy has reduced the rates of thyroid surgery in patients with nodular thyroid disease by approximately 25% and doubled the rate of thyroid cancer in patients undergoing thyroid surgery [102, 103]. The procedure is safe, inexpensive, accurate and can be performed in the office. Complications such as hematoma or severe pain are uncommon, and the false positive and false negative rates are very low [104].

Compared to FNA by palpation, UG-FNA of the thyroid has greater sensitivity, specificity and accuracy, especially for non-palpable and posterior nodules, mixed

Samer El-Kaissi & Jack R Wall

predominantly cystic nodules, and previously sampled nodules by palpation with a non-diagnostic FNA [35]. UG-FNA has been shown to decrease the incidence of inadequate specimens from 15% by palpation to less than 3% [105, 106], and to reduce the risk of false negative specimens by ensuring that suspicious thyroid lesions are biopsied [107]. The use of Rapid on-site cytological Evaluation (ROSE) may further improve specimen adequacy [108].

Before performing an UG-FNA, a detailed thyroid ultrasound scan provides information about the nodule(s) that warrant FNA based on malignancy risk stratification and nodule size, the location and character of the nodule(s), and whether there is any suspicious cervical lymphadenopathy that may require evaluation by FNA. The baseline ultrasound also allows selection of an appropriate entry angle and path in order to avoid vital structures in the neck.

After explaining the benefits and risks of the UG-FNA procedure to the patient and obtaining an informed consent, the patient is positioned supine with the neck extended comfortably in the same position as that for the thyroid ultrasound examination. The degree of neck extension may be limited in patients with osteoarthritis of the cervical spine so that the degree of neck extension should be adjusted to keep the patient as comfortable as possible. It is preferable to have the ultrasound monitor facing the physician or above the patient's head so that the physician does not need to look away from the patient during the procedure. A small amount of gel is smeared onto the foot of the transducer before applying a latex probe cover.

In an aseptic technique, the skin is cleansed and alcohol or sterile water is used as a coupling agent during the procedure. The patient is warned that the procedure is about to start and asked to keep still and to avoid swallowing if possible. The skin is punctured rather quickly to minimize discomfort and the needle is then advanced slowly under ultrasound guidance towards the target. Once the bevel of the needle is visualized within the target, the bevel is gently advanced and withdrawn repeatedly from the proximal edge to the distal edge of the lesion and with every advancement, the needle is slightly rotated clock-wise allowing the sharp bevel to cut cells into the lumen of the needle. This technique is preferred to a rapid up and down jabbing motion that requires great care to prevent the needle from exiting the target lesion [107]. For large superficial nodules, slight alteration of the needle angle after withdrawal to the periphery of the target lesion allows sampling different areas of the nodule as demonstrated in Fig. (**6**). This manoeuvre is best avoided for deep-seated nodules as the tip of the needle cannot be withdrawn sufficiently to change the angle.

Subsequently, the needle is rapidly withdrawn and an assistant applies gentle pressure to the biopsy site for 1-2 minutes. With every subsequent pass, a different area of the lesion is biopsied and in most cases two passes are adequate, but more passes are occasionally required which is where ROSE becomes invaluable. While many physicians prefer to apply negative pressure during the procedure either with a syringe holder or a 'gun', allowing the biopsy material to enter the needle by capillary action, known as 'capillary FNA', is equally effective and may be associated with a lower rate of bloody aspirates [109, 110]. Although no longer in production, the Tao syringe holder applies suction through a spring-loaded mechanism. Because it is difficult to control the negative pressure during withdrawal of the needle, biopsy material may end up being wasted in the barrel of the syringe.

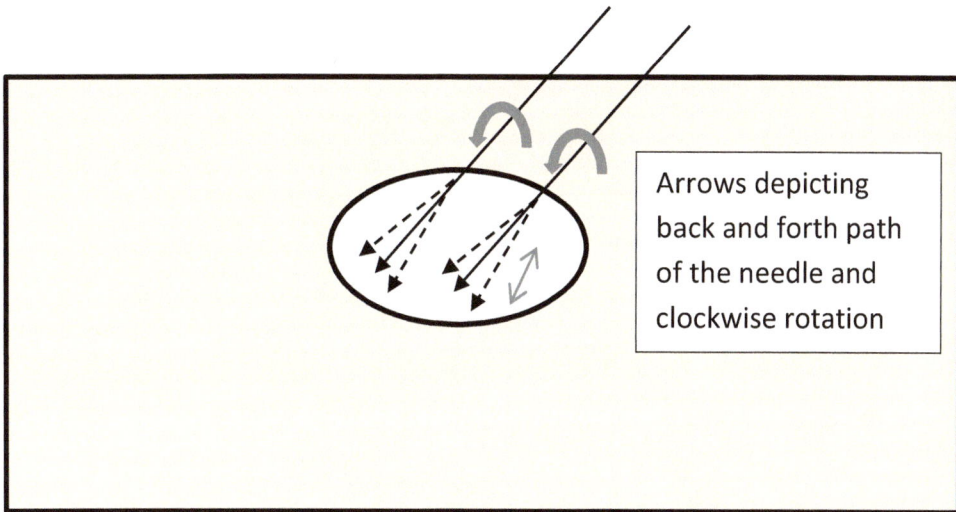

Fig. (6). FNA biopsy of a thyroid nodule under ultrasound guidance. A minimum of 2 passes is performed on each nodule, moving the bevel of the needle back and forth within the nodule with slight clockwise rotation while advancing the needle. Whenever possible, the bevel of the needle is withdrawn to the superficial border of the nodule and the angle of the needle is gently adjusted to sample a wider area of the nodule.

The needle path is either parallel or perpendicular to the ultrasound beam. With the perpendicular approach, the needle is inserted at the centre of the long axis of the transducer foot and is angled slightly towards the transducer, whereas in the parallel approach the needle is inserted at the centre of the short axis of the transducer foot. Turning the bevel of the needle up towards the ultrasound beam allows greater visibility of the needle tip during the procedure. Compared to the perpendicular approach, the parallel approach is probably safer as it allows visualization of the whole needle throughout the procedure but requires more practice and uses up more needle length. It is ideal for more superficial nodules that are in close proximity to vital structures in the neck, for aspiration of cystic nodules and for percutaneous ethanol injection (PEI). A needle guide that attaches to the transducer shows the proposed needle path on the monitor and can be useful until the physician becomes more comfortable with the parallel approach. With the perpendicular approach, only the bevel of the needle can be seen and this approach is best reserved for deeper thyroid nodules that are not in close proximity to vital structures in the neck [107].

Most nodules can be easily sampled with a 1.5" needle length. For solid nodules, 25-27G needles are often sufficient whereas a larger gauge needle (22-24G) is required for the aspiration of cystic content. Attaching the needle to a 10 cc syringe allows greater manoeuvrability of the needle and is essential for aspiration during the procedure. Before the procedure, the syringe is pre-filled with 1-2 cc of air in preparation for the expulsion of the aspirate onto slides after the biopsy. For capillary FNA, the plunger is best removed from the syringe. Drainage of large cystic thyroid nodules can be performed by attaching the biopsy needle to a connecting tube with a syringe at the other end. While the sonographer positions the needle at the centre of the cyst, an assistant aspirates the cyst contents.

For patient comfort, it is generally recommended to limit FNA biopsy to 2 nodules per visit. Nodules that do not meet the size cut-off criteria for FNA biopsy are best observed with serial ultrasound, but occasionally smaller nodules could be biopsied if there is a high suspicion for malignancy on ultrasound, evidence of ETE or suspicious CLNs, or if there is a personal or family history of thyroid cancer or recent onset dysphonia [111].

For heterogeneous nodules, the biopsy specimen should be taken from the more suspicious part of the nodule such as a hypoechoic region or an area displaying microcalcifications (Image **29**). When multiple nodules are present, it is important to select nodules with suspicious ultrasonographic characteristics for FNA biopsy regardless of nodule size. If all the nodules display similar ultrasound features, one could biopsy the dominant nodule in each thyroid lobe [35].

Depending on patient preference, subcutaneous local anaesthesia can be used to reduce discomfort at the skin puncture site. FNA biopsy of CLNs follows the same principle as FNA biopsy of a thyroid. Briefly, a 25-27G needle is advanced into the CLN under US-guidance in a perpendicular or parallel approach to the long axis of the transducer. Both capillary and aspiration techniques are acceptable.

While the risk of bleeding post-FNA biopsy is very low (less than 1%), a haematoma can be avoided by minimizing the number of passes, applying gentle compression at the biopsy site after each pass, and performing a brief ultrasound scan of the biopsy site at the end of the procedure (Image **36**). The patient is advised to report severe neck discomfort or swelling that may occur within 24-hours after the procedure. There are no prospective studies in patients taking antithrombotic medications which include anticoagulants and antiplatelet agents, and a retrospective study found no increase in the risk of bleeding in 144 patients on antithrombotic or anticoagulant medications who underwent UG-FNA biopsy of neck lesions compared to patients not taking these medications [112].

However, the American Association of Clinical Endocrinologists (AACE) guidelines recommend whenever possible to discontinue antithrombotic agents for 3-5 days before the FNA procedure and anticoagulant medications before 5 days [111]. If necessary, oral anticoagulant therapy can be substituted with low-molecular weight heparin which is withheld 24 hours before the procedure. Compared to warfarin, novel oral anticoagulants (NOACs) have a much shorter half-life and can be withheld 24 hours before the procedure. Whether or not antithrombotic therapies are withheld before the procedure, it is important to follow the principles described above to minimize the risk of bleeding and to ensure that in patients taking warfarin the international normalized ratio (INR) is less than 2.5-3.0 before the procedure [86].

The FNA biopsy material is deposited onto a pre-labelled slide. Cytopathology slides can be prepared using either the classic three slides or two-slide 'book-end' techniques [113]. Both methods produce two slides, the first slide is quickly fixed in 95% alcohol for Papanicolaou staining and the second slide is air-dried in preparation for staining with Diff-Quik, a commercial Romanowsky stain variant. More information on slide preparation and staining can be found in Reference [114]. It is essential to note that slide preparation and staining is largely based on the preference of the cytopathologist.

After preparing the slides, the needle is rinsed in Cytolyt solution which is used to create a ThinPrep slide or a cell block if necessary. The exclusive use of liquid-based biopsies and ThinPrep is emerging as an alternative to traditional cytopathology slides [115, 116]. Depending on the clinical scenario, the needle can be rinsed in 1-ml normal saline for measurement of biomarkers such as thyroglobulin (FNA-Tg; see Ultrasound in Thyroid Cancer Surveillance Section), calcitonin (FNA-calcitonin) or parathyroid hormone (FNA-PTH). Genetic markers such as BRAF and TERT gene mutations can also be assessed on FNA material if clinically indicated [117, 118].

Thyroid nodule and cervical node FNA-calcitonin can be measured in patients with suspected MTC especially in those with elevated serum calcitonin. In one study, thyroid nodule FNA-calcitonin greater than 1000 pg/mL was diagnostic of MTC, whereas levels between 36-1000 pg/mL were indeterminate [119]. In another study, FNA-calcitonin levels up to 67 pg/mL were seen in benign thyroid nodules [120]. Boi *et al.* [121] found that CLN and thyroid nodule FNA calcitonin levels greater than 36 pg/mL had 100% sensitivity and specificity for the diagnosis of MTC compared to standard cytopathology which had a sensitivity of 62% and specificity of 80%. Despite the disagreement on the FNA-calcitonin cut-off for the diagnosis of MTC, the test is still quite useful as most patients with MTC have FNA-calcitonin that is much higher than the serum calcitonin.

Given the high diagnostic rates of parathyroidectomy, FNA biopsies of suspected parathyroid adenomas are not routinely required and are reserved for cases with discrepant neck imaging and for patients with persistent hyperparathyroidism post-surgical exploration. A FNA-PTH level greater than the serum PTH is suggestive of a parathyroid lesion. In one study, FNA-PTH out-performed standard cytopathology which had a poor sensitivity of 40% and a high non-diagnostic rate at 28% [122].

Many thyroid centres are now using the Bethesda System for Reporting Thyroid Cytopathology (BSRTC) [123, 124] which consists of six diagnostic categories, although some centres in Europe and the Middle East prefer the UK Royal College of Pathologists grading system [shown in square brackets]:

  I. Non-diagnostic/unsatisfactory [Thyroid 1]
 II. Benign [Thyroid 2]
III. Atypia of undetermined significance (AUS)/follicular lesion of undetermined significance (FLUS) [Thyroid 3a]
IV. Follicular neoplasm (FN)/suspicious for follicular neoplasm (SFN) [Thyroid 3f]
 V. Suspicious for malignancy (SUSP) [Thyroid 4]
VI. Malignant [Thyroid 5]

Based on a meta-analysis of 8 studies [125], the actual risk of malignancy of Bethesda categories I-VI is 16.8%, 3.7%, 15.9%, 26.1%, 75.2% and 98.6%, respectively. One limitation of these studies is selection bias, as patients with sonographically worrisome nodules and clinical risk factors for thyroid malignancy are preferentially referred for thyroidectomy. This leads to an increased risk of malignancy in patients with Bethesda categories I, III, IV and V, and it has been suggested that the estimated risk of malignancy for each Bethesda category may be more accurate [124]. Furthermore, the actual risk of malignancy includes patients with non-invasive follicular thyroid neoplasm with papillary-like nuclear features (NIFTP) which is likely overestimating the risk of malignancy. The estimated risk ranges of malignancy for Bethesda I-VI are 5-10%, 0-3%, 6-18%, 10-40%, 45-60% and 94-96% respectively when NIFTP is not counted as a malignancy, and 5-10%, 0-3%, 10-30%, 25-40%, 50-75% and 97-99% when NIFTP is included [124].

The use of BSRTC may increase the rate of indeterminate thyroid nodules [126], but its widespread adoption is expected to bring uniformity and consistency in thyroid cytopathology reporting. Because of significant variations in the risk of malignancy of each of the diagnostic categories between different centres, especially for Bethesda categories III, IV and V (indeterminate cytopathology), it is recommended that clinical centres determine their own risk of malignancy associated with each Bethesda category.

CHAPTER 7

Clinical Management of Thyroid Nodules

Abstract: The management of thyroid nodules begins with a detailed ultrasound examination to document the size and ultrasound features of the nodule and thereby determine the risk malignancy. In hyperthyroid patients, a thyroid scintigram is important as the great majority of hyperfunctioning thyroid nodules are benign. Depending on the ultrasound pattern and size of the nodule, FNA biopsy may be clinically indicated to exclude malignancy. A benign FNA biopsy completes the diagnostic workup, however ongoing monitoring and repeat FNA biopsy may be warranted in nodules displaying a high suspicion of malignancy on ultrasound. Non-diagnostic nodules should undergo repeat FNA biopsy under ultrasound guidance and if persistently non-diagnostic, management options include observation of very low to low-suspicion nodules and thyroid surgery for nodules with an intermediate or high suspicion pattern on ultrasound. Indeterminate nodules (Bethesda III, IV and V) require further diagnostic workup and/or thyroidectomy. While Bethesda IV and V nodules are primarily treated surgically, our approach is to repeat the FNA biopsy with/without molecular testing for Bethesda III nodules and to consider ongoing observation or thyroid surgery for persistently indeterminate nodules, depending on the sonographic and cytological suspicion of malignancy. Cytologically malignant nodules are also referred for thyroidectomy. The extent of thyroid surgery depends on the size of the thyroid nodule, the patient's clinical risk factors for thyroid malignancy, the risk of extra-thyroidal extension and patient preference.

Keywords: Atypia of undetermined significance, Benign cytology, Bethesda system for reporting thyroid cytopathology, Core-needle biopsy, FNA biopsy, Follicular lesion of undetermined significance, Follicular neoplasm, Indeterminate cytology, Non-diagnostic cytology, Suspicious for malignancy, Thyroid nodule, Thyroid malignancy, Thyroid nodule molecular testing, Thyroidectomy, Thyroid nodule growth, Thyroid nodule follow-up.

Following the discovery of thyroid nodule(s) on ultrasound, plasma TSH is measured and if low, or low-normal in a multinodular goitre, thyroid scintigraphy is performed to identify hot nodules which are most likely benign. Patients with a low plasma TSH and cold nodules on scintigraphy, and patients with a non-suppressed plasma TSH are managed according to the nodules' risk of malignancy and specific nodule size cut-offs on ultrasound (Fig. **7**). Measurement

Samer El-Kaissi & Jack R Wall

of plasma thyroglobulin is unhelpful in discriminating benign from malignant thyroid nodules, while plasma calcitonin could be considered in cases of suspected MTC. An unstimulated plasma calcitonin above 50 pg/ml is suggestive of MTC [35].

For nodules with a clinical indication for FNA biopsy, future management and follow-up are dictated by the cytopathology result as reported by the BSRTC (Table **9**, Fig. **7**).

Bethesda I: A non-diagnostic or unsatisfactory diagnosis (Bethesda category I) is seen in up to 20% of FNA biopsies because of insufficient follicular cells. In one study, the rate of malignancy in non-diagnostic nodules with suspicious features on ultrasound was as high as 25%, compared to 4% in nodules with low suspicion features [127]. Non-diagnostic nodules should be followed-up initially with a repeat UG-FNA biopsy unless the nodule has a very low suspicion for thyroid malignancy, in which case observation is a valid option. Delaying the repeat FNA by approximately 3-months from the original aspiration was reported to reduce the risk of false positive cytopathology [128], but these findings were not supported in two subsequent studies [129, 130]. The repeat FNA is diagnostic in up to 80% of cases, especially if the cystic component is less than 50% [131, 132]. Persistently non-diagnostic nodules with benign or very low suspicion of malignancy on ultrasound may be observed with periodical ultrasound scans, whereas nodules associated with clinical risk factors for malignancy, suspicious ultrasound characteristics and an interval increase in size during follow-up may warrant surgical intervention. The role of molecular testing and core-needle biopsy (CNB) has not been elucidated in repeatedly non-diagnostic thyroid nodules. CNB may provide better adequacy but is less sensitive than FNA for the diagnosis of PTC [133, 134].

Bethesda II: Nodules with a benign FNA have a very small risk of malignancy and require no further diagnostic workup unless the nodule has a high suspicion for malignancy on ultrasound. In such cases, repeating the thyroid ultrasound and FNA within 6-months is advised. The risk of malignancy in cytologically benign nodules is less than 3% and close to 0% in nodules with two benign biopsies [135 - 137]. It is not clear if nodules larger than 3-4 cm should be managed differently due to reports of higher rates of malignancy and false negative FNA [82, 138 - 140], especially because these concerns were not confirmed in other studies [83, 141].

This algorithm can be used with other thyroid nodule ultrasound risk stratification systems such as the European Thyroid Association TI-RADS (Table 5) and the American College of Radiology TI-RADS (Table 6) after accounting for differences in FNA biopsy cut-offs. Dotted arrows depict alternative management pathways. Adapted from reference [32] with permission.

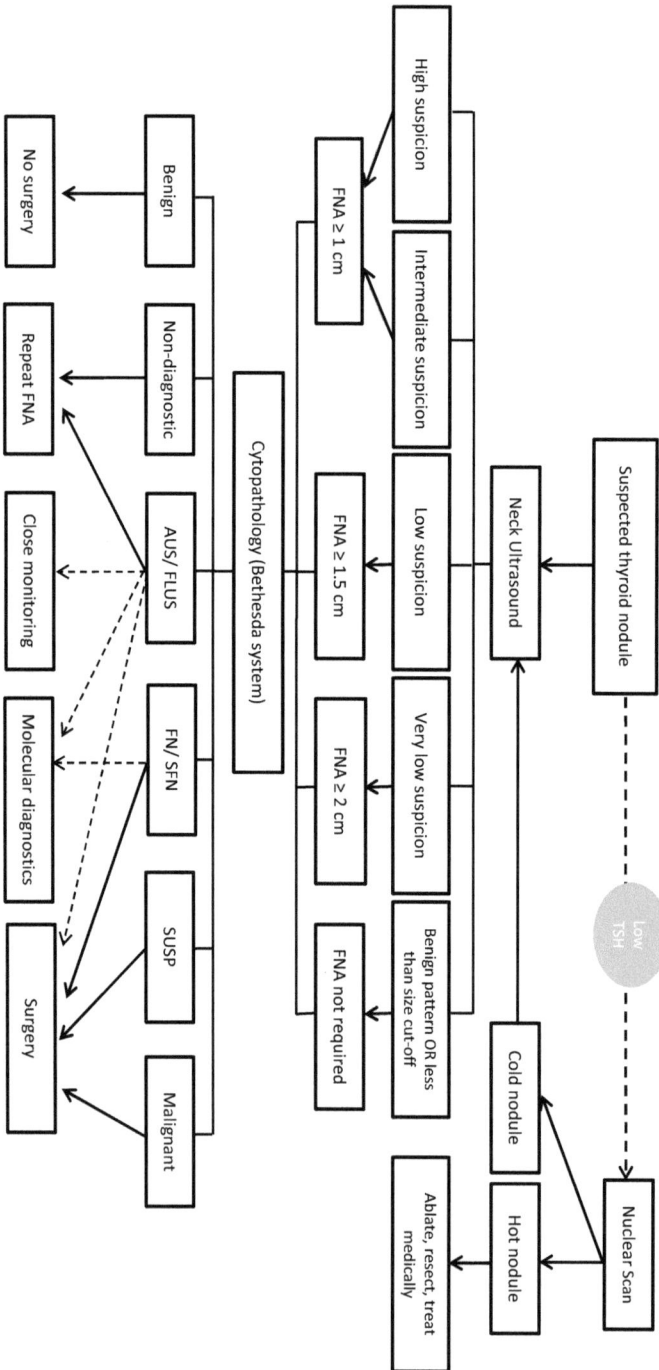

Fig. (7). Thyroid nodule management algorithm based on the American Thyroid Association 2015 Guidelines for the management of thyroid nodules.

Bethesda III: Up to one-third of thyroid nodule FNAs are reported as indeterminate [125], thereby requiring further diagnostic workup. AUS/FLUS constitute architectural and/or nuclear atypia on cytology, with nuclear atypia carrying a greater potential for malignancy. While the estimated risk of malignancy in these nodules does not exceed 20%, there is significant variability between cytopathology centres, and nodules with a high suspicion pattern on ultrasound have a much higher risk of malignancy, reaching up to 90% in some studies [142, 143]. Nevertheless, in many AUS/FLUS cases the cytology sample is of borderline adequacy and repeating the FNA biopsy under ultrasound guidance provides a conclusive diagnosis in up to 70% of cases [144, 145]. One study questioned the value of repeat FNA biopsy in Bethesda III nodules due to the persistently increased risk of malignancy of a nodule with an initial AUS diagnosis and a subsequent benign cytopathology (2/7 cases; 29%), although the small sample size may have contributed to these findings [146]. Our approach is to repeat FNA biopsy with/without molecular testing for Bethesda III nodules. In repeatedly cytologically indeterminate nodules, we offer patients with very low to low-suspicion features on ultrasound and predominantly architectural atypia continued observation, while patients harbouring nodules with nuclear atypia and/or intermediate to high suspicion features on ultrasound are referred for a surgical opinion. The is an increasing number of molecular tests for thyroid nodules on the market, including the 167-gene expression classifier (Afirma) and next-generation mutational sequencing panels (ThyroSeq v3). Limitations of these molecular tests are cost and the lack of long-term studies supporting their clinical utility. The role of core-needle biopsy in this setting remains to be determined but seems promising [147].

Bethesda IV: The estimated risk of malignancy in these nodules can reach 40% and our approach is to consider surgery, usually without any further diagnostic workup. However, after taking into account the ultrasound features of the nodule, the patient's clinical risk factors for thyroid malignancy and the patient's preference, molecular testing may be considered.

Bethesda V: the risk of malignancy exceeds 50% in these nodules and patients should be referred for a surgical opinion.

Bethesda VI: The risk of a false positive FNA is less than 3% and all patients with malignant cytology are referred for thyroid surgery. The extent of thyroid surgery depends on the clinical risk factors for thyroid malignancy, size of the tumour, the presence of extra-thyroidal extension and patient preference.

The 2015 ATA guidelines provide follow-up recommendations for thyroid nodules based primarily on the ultrasound suspicion of malignancy (Table **10**)

[35]. Regardless of whether thyroid nodule FNA biopsy was previously performed and reported as benign, UG-FNA biopsy at the time of follow-up thyroid ultrasound should be considered for sonographically high suspicion nodules, and for other nodules displaying a significant increase in size and new suspicious features on ultrasound. It is important to note that nodule growth on ultrasound is not associated with malignancy in the absence of suspicious sonographic features [135, 148], and routine monitoring of nodule growth to predict malignancy was not justified in a meta-analysis of more than 2700 patients [149]. After two benign FNAs, the risk of malignancy is negligible and ongoing follow-up for malignancy is unlikely to be beneficial, although many patients require follow-up for nodule size and for the development of neck compressive symptoms. Similarly, subcentimetric nodules with very low suspicion for malignancy on ultrasound are unlikely to change significantly over the next 5 years and follow-up can be discontinued [150].

Table 9. The Bethesda System for Reporting Thyroid Cytopathology and the recommended clinical management for each category based on the 2015 American Thyroid Association Guidelines for the management of thyroid nodules [35]. Thyroidectomy may be partial or complete depending on the clinical risk factors, size of the tumour, likelihood of extra-thyroidal extension and patient preference. CNB – core needle biopsy.

Diagnosis	Bethesda Category	Management
Non-diagnostic or unsatisfactory	I	Repeat FNA under ultrasound guidance, consider CNB and thyroidectomy
Benign	II	Monitor
Atypia of undetermined significance (AUS)/ Follicular lesion of undetermined significance (FLUS)	III	Repeat FNA Consider molecular testing and/or thyroidectomy
Follicular neoplasm (FN) or suspicious for a follicular neoplasm (SFN)	IV	Thyroidectomy Consider molecular testing
Suspicious for malignancy (SUSP)	V	Thyroidectomy
Malignant	VI	Thyroidectomy

Table 10. Follow-up of thyroid nodules is based on the suspicion of malignancy on ultrasound [35].

Suspicion of malignancy on ultrasound	Follow-up thyroid Ultrasound (months)
High	6-12
Low to intermediate	12-24
Very low	> 24

CHAPTER 8

Ultrasound in Thyroid Cancer Surveillance

Abstract: Plasma thyroglobulin and neck ultrasound allow the detection of residual or recurrent disease in the majority of post-operative differentiated thyroid cancer patients. The two tests are complimentary to each other and are better than either test alone. Neck ultrasound is superior to neck palpation and allows morphological differentiation of benign from suspicious cervical lymph nodes. A baseline neck ultrasound is performed at 3-6 months post-operatively to examine the neck for persistent thyroid cancer and to plan for radioactive iodine ablation in patients at an increased risk for thyroid cancer recurrence. Neck ultrasonography is repeated periodically thereafter to exclude recurrent disease. Suspicious cervical lymph nodes and thyroid bed lesions can be biopsied under ultrasound guidance, and a needle washout obtained for measurement of thyroglobulin in patients with differentiated thyroid cancer and calcitonin in medullary thyroid cancer. Neck ultrasound also allows the examination of other anterior neck structures such as muscle and blood vessels for invasive disease and can be used to mark the location of suspicious nodes pre- or intra-operatively. In patients with elevated plasma tumour markers and negative neck ultrasound, whole body iodine scan or cross-sectional imaging may be useful.

Keywords: Anti-thyroglobulin antibody, Clinical neck palpation, Calcitonin, Cytopathology, Metastatic cervical lymph node, Neck ultrasound, Positron emission tomography, Recurrence of differentiated thyroid cancer, Thyroidectomy, Thyroid cancer, Thyroglobulin, Thyroid bed, Thyroid tissue remnant, Whole body iodine scan, Whole body single photon emission tomography.

Following thyroid surgery for DTC, the combination of neck ultrasonography and serum thyroglobulin are an excellent tool for the detection of recurrent disease, with positive and negative predictive values approaching 100%, and are more accurate than either method alone [151, 152]. However, serum thyroglobulin may be falsely normal in patients with elevated anti-thyroglobulin antibodies and is less useful than ultrasound post-lobectomy. Furthermore, neck ultrasonography should precede the measurement of a TSH-stimulated thyroglobulin as up to 18% of DTC patients with CLN recurrence on ultrasound have a stimulated serum thyroglobulin less than 1.0 ng/mL [152].

In patients with recurrent DTC post-operatively, neck ultrasonography returns positive findings in up to 96% of cases and is superior to clinical palpation which detects less than 18% of neck lesions especially because around half of the recurrent lesions are less than 1 cm in size [152 - 154]. Neck ultrasound is also ideal for post-operative cancer surveillance because approximately 75% of recurrences are seen in the anterior CLNs and 20% are found in the thyroid bed [155]. Ultrasound has an added advantage over other imaging modalities in its ability to morphologically differentiate benign CLN from those with suspicious features.

An initial neck ultrasound is performed 3-6 months post-thyroidectomy to assess for the presence of persistent disease and help in the planning for radioactive iodine ablation if clinically indicated. Care should be taken not to perform the thyroid ultrasound in the immediate post-operative period to avoid the detection of post-operative changes that may be falsely interpreted as positive findings (Image **45**). This is particularly important as many centres are using Surgicel which mimics thyroid tissue on ultrasound and can take 8 weeks or longer to be completely resorbed [156]. A second scan is obtained at 6-12 months to assess for recurrence and yearly thereafter for up to 5 years post-operatively for patients at intermediate or high risk of recurrence. After 5 years, most patients can be followed with serum thyroglobulin and anti-thyroglobulin antibodies. However, patients with abnormal scans, persistent/recurrent disease or rising plasma thyroglobulin and/or anti-thyroglobulin antibody levels may benefit from more frequent neck scans *e.g.* every 6-months, depending on their TNM stage and risk of recurrence. Patients at low risk for tumour recurrence who have a normal scan at 6-months post-operatively do not require an annual neck ultrasound. Post-lobectomy, an initial neck ultrasound is obtained at 6-12 months and if normal, every 2-3 years thereafter [86].

The post-operative neck ultrasound examination begins in the thyroid bed (Image **44**), an inverted hyperechoic triangular area [157] that represents postoperative fibro-fatty changes, and any suspicious lesions are characterized and measured. Isoechoic or slightly hypoechoic, ovoid lesions in the thyroid bed often represent thyroid tissue remnants (Image **47**) whereas hypoechoic lesions that are darker than the strap muscles may be due to persistent or recurrent DTC (Image **46**), especially if associated with microcalcifications, cystic component, irregular margins, increased vascularity or taller than wide shape in the transverse plane [157 - 159]. Apart from thyroid remnants and recurrent disease, the differential diagnosis for hypoechoic lesions in the thyroid bed includes central CLNs and parathyroid adenomas [86]. Less commonly, other structures may be mistaken for thyroid bed lesions. These include the thyroid and cricoid cartilage, cervical thymus and cervical sympathetic ganglia [156].

Examination of the thyroid bed is followed by a detailed examination of the anterior CLN as described in Chapter IV: Ultrasound of cervical lymph nodes. Any suspicious nodes are examined using grey-scale and Doppler study, their location documented and size is measured in 3-dimensions. Structures that may mimic nodal disease in the neck include the thoracic duct, TGD cysts, cervical nerve roots, and degenerative changes of the sternoclavicular joints [156]. It is also important to briefly examine the anterior neck muscles and the great vessels of the neck especially the internal jugular vein (Image **48**) for tumour thrombi or invasion [160, 161]. Tumour invasion or recurrence in surrounding muscle tissue appears on ultrasound as a solid mass with irregular margins and increased vascularity [86].

When clinically indicated, suspicious thyroid bed lesions and cervical nodes greater than 8-10 mm in their smallest dimension can be further evaluated with UG-FNA biopsies and FNA-Tg with a high degree of accuracy [35]. Following preparation of cytology slides, FNA-Tg is collected by rinsing the needle in 1 ml normal saline and thyroglobulin is measured using an immunometric assay calibrated against the Certified Reference Material 457 [CRM-457], an international human thyroglobulin reference standard, with a 0.1-1.0 µg/L functional sensitivity of the assay. FNA-Tg improves the sensitivity and NPV of CLN cytopathology which may be non-diagnostic in 5-10% of cases, falsely negative in 6-8% of patients [162] and can yield a false positive result in another 6-8% of cases [163 - 165]. FNA-Tg may be most useful for cystic CLN that often have low cellularity [86].

A cervical node FNA-Tg greater than 10 ng/mL is consistent with nodal metastasis, whereas FNA-Tg 1-10 ng/mL confers a moderate suspicion for malignancy and levels less than 1 ng/mL are interpreted as negative for malignancy [35]. It has been suggested that the actual concentration of thyroglobulin in the CLN (ng/mL) may be inaccurate as it does not take into account the dilutional factor [86]. Some investigators advocate using the concentration of thyroglobulin per FNA pass in 1 ml normal saline as a more accurate measure of FNA-Tg with cut off values less than 1 ng/FNA as normal, 1-10 ng/FNA as indeterminate and greater than 10 ng/FNA as positive for malignancy [166]. FNA-Tg is correlated with serum TSH and thyroglobulin levels [167], but whether positive anti-thyroglobulin antibodies lead to false lowering of FNA-Tg remains controversial [35, 168]. In patients with a history of MTC, FNA-calcitonin can be very useful when the cytopathology is inconclusive or non-diagnostic (see Chapter VI. Ultrasound-Guided Fine Needle Aspiration Biopsy).

For the surgical resection of metastatic CLNs, several techniques are available to help the surgeon localize pathological nodes in the neck. The use of neck ultrasound on the day of surgery to localize and mark the skin over the area of recurrence allows resection of lesions as small as 6 mm and reduces the risk of operative failure [169]. Pre-operative intra-nodal injection of charcoal suspension under ultrasound guidance lasts more than 3 months but may leave a skin mark at the injection site [86]. Alternatively, intra-operative labelling of malignant lesions in the neck with methylene blue under ultrasound guidance has been advocated by some clinicians [170].

Patients with sonographically suspicious thyroid bed lesions and CLNs that are smaller than 8 mm can be observed with serial neck ultrasound *e.g.* every 6-12 months, and FNA biopsy is performed if the lesion is increasing in size. This approach seems reasonable as malignant lateral neck nodes remain stable for a long time [171], and biochemical remission post-surgical excision of malignant nodes does not exceed 27% [172].

In patients with a persistently elevated serum thyroglobulin and negative neck ultrasound, other imaging modalities such as a whole body iodine scan, whole body single photon emission tomography-CT (SPECT-CT) and positron emission tomography-CT (PET-CT) are valuable tools to exclude the presence of distant metastases.

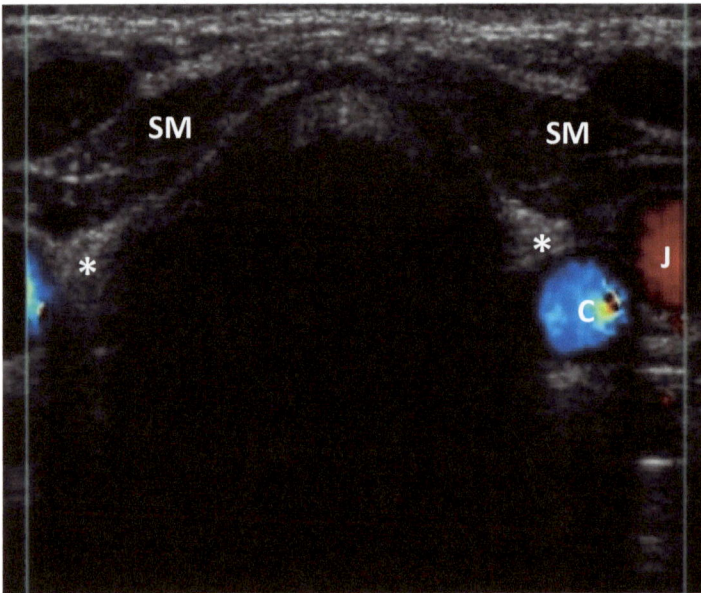

Image (44). Thyroid bed, transverse plane, post-total thyroidectomy for papillary thyroid carcinoma demonstrating post-operative fibro-fatty changes (*) with no residual thyroid tissue. C = carotid artery, J = internal jugular vein, SM = strap muscles of the neck.

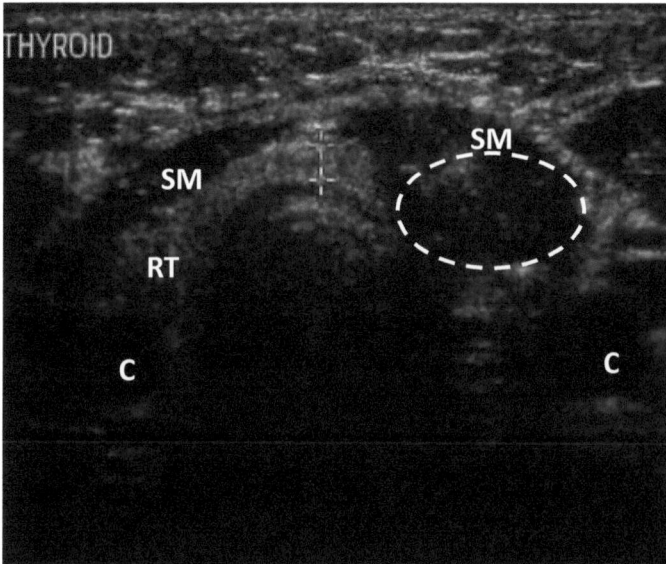

Image (45). Left hemithyroidectomy for papillary thyroid carcinoma. Note absence of the left thyroid lobe with an intact isthmus and right thyroid lobe (RT). Fullness of the left thyroid bed (circle) rather than the typical collapsed appearance is due to post-operative changes as the scan was performed less than 1-month post-operatively. It is best to delay neck ultrasound for a few months after thyroidectomy to allow post-operative changes to settle. C = carotid artery, SM = strap muscles of the neck.

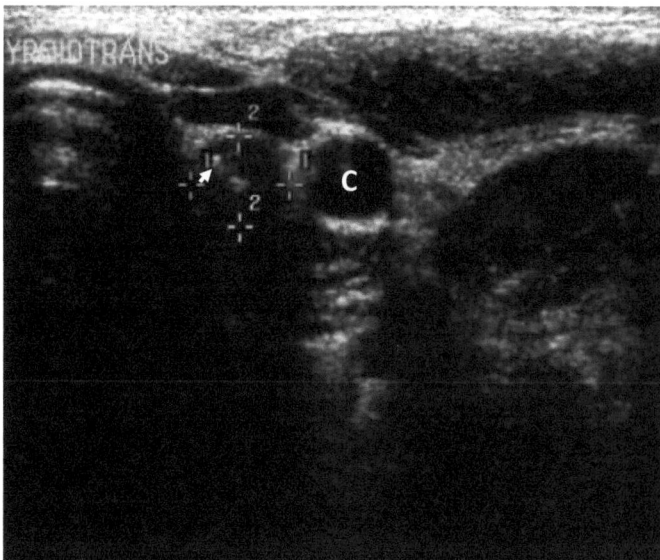

Image (46). Left thyroid bed tumour recurrence post-total thyroidectomy for papillary thyroid carcinoma. There is a hypoechoic focus with irregular margins and calcifications (arrow) in the left thyroid bed. FNA biopsy of this mass with measurement of thyroglobulin in the biopsy needle washout confirmed the diagnosis of recurrent papillary thyroid carcinoma. C = carotid artery.

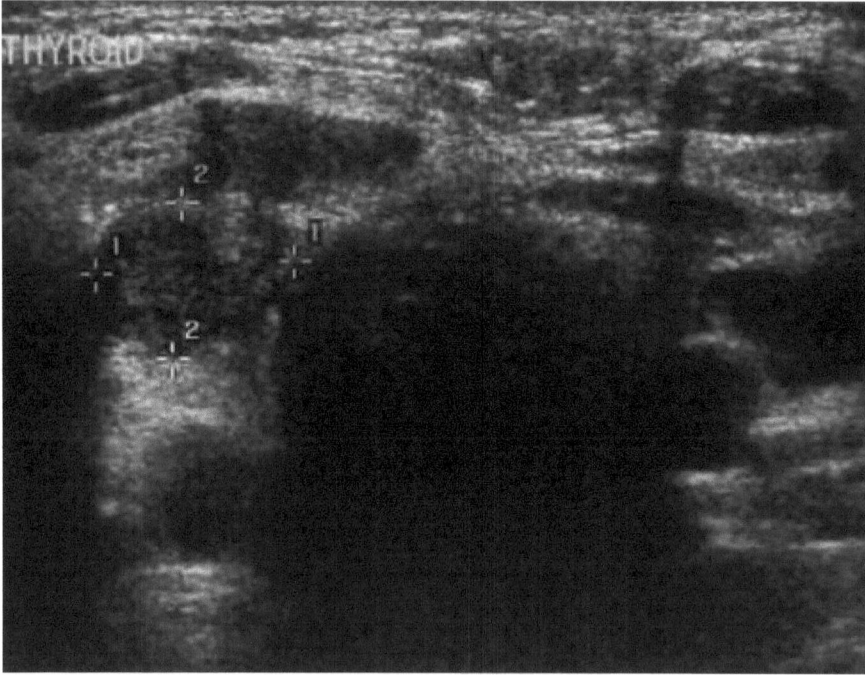

Image (47). Right thyroid bed mass, transverse plane, post-total thyroidectomy in a patient with papillary thyroid carcinoma. The mass has regular margins with no calcifications or cystic changes. FNA biopsy of this mass can help differentiate benign thyroid tissue remnants from recurrent disease.

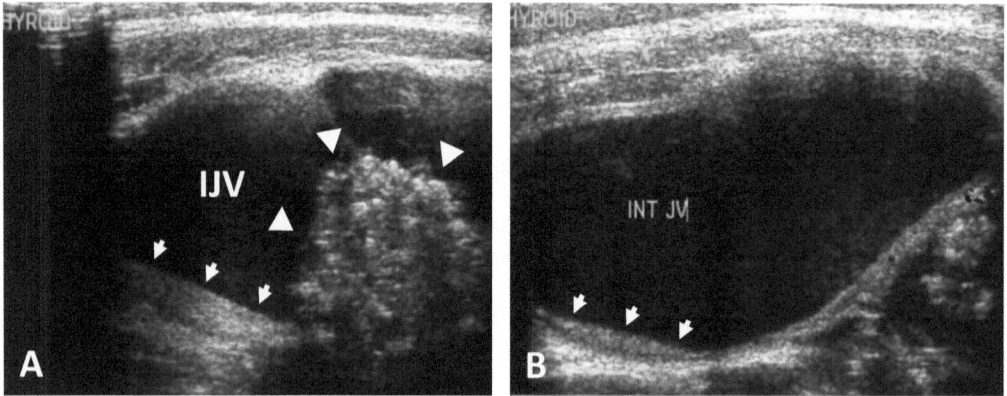

Image (48). Dilated right internal jugular vein (IJV) with a calcific mass invading into the vein (arrowheads, A). The IJV was thrombosed at the site of the tumour with no demonstrable flow on Doppler (B) and a fluid level can be seen (arrows). The patient has a history of an untreated 5 cm right lobe papillary thyroid carcinoma.

CHAPTER 9

Ultrasound in Autoimmune Thyroid Disease

Abstract: Autoimmune thyroid disease is a common thyroid disorder that encompasses a number of conditions including Hashimoto's thyroiditis, atrophic thyroiditis and Graves' disease. Hashimoto's thyroiditis presents on ultrasound as a hypoechoic, heterogeneous and asymmetrical thyroid gland. Other sonographic features of Hashimoto's thyroiditis are micronodulation, fibrous bands, pseudonodules, hyperechoic regenerative thyroid nodules, and cervical lymphadenopathy especially in the central compartment. The ultrasound features of Graves' disease are less marked than Hashimoto's thyroiditis and include a diffuse goitre with reduced thyroid gland echogenicity and increased vascularity on Doppler study. The presence of thyroid nodules in hyperthyroid Graves' patients requires further evaluation with thyroid ultrasound, thyroid scintigraphy and FNA biopsy of any suspicious and hypofunctioning nodules. Subacute (De Quervain's) thyroiditis most probably has a viral aetiology and patients present with a tender thyroid gland and raised inflammatory markers. The thyroid gland displays hypoechoic areas with reduced Doppler flow on ultrasound. On the other hand silent thyroiditis and its variant, post-partum thyroiditis, present on thyroid ultrasound as a slightly hypoechoic and heterogeneous gland. There are two types of amiodarone-induced hyperthyroidism, type 1 which resembles Graves' disease with increased vascularity on Doppler study and type 2 disease that is associated with destructive thyroiditis and normal or reduced vascularity.

Keywords: Autoimmune thyroid disease, Atrophic thyroiditis, Amiodarone-induced hyperthyroidism, Cervical lymphadenoathy, Fibrous bands, Graves' disease, Hashimoto's thyroiditis, Heterogeneous, Hypoechoic, Micronodulation, Post-partum thyroiditis, Pseudonodules, Regenerative hyperechoic nodules, Silent thyroiditis, Subacute thyroiditis, Thyroid inferno, Ultrasound Doppler study.

Autoimmune thyroid disease (AITD) deserves a special mention as it is relatively common, alters the sonographic architecture of the thyroid gland, and displays specific features on ultrasound. AITD is a general term that encompasses a number of thyroid conditions, the hallmark of which is an increase in one or more of the thyroid autoantibodies and thyroid dysfunction. These conditions include Hashimoto's (HT) and atrophic thyroiditis, Graves' disease (GD) and a small subset (25-30%) of patients with painless thyroiditis and post-partum thyroiditis.

Samer El-Kaissi & Jack R Wall

HT presents clinically with an asymmetrical goitre in contrast to atrophic thyroiditis, where the thyroid gland is shrunken and difficult to palpate. HT and atrophic thyroiditis are often associated with hypothyroidism, elevated anti-thyroid peroxidase antibodies (TPO-Ab) and anti-thyroglobulin antibodies although only TPO-Ab have been associated with the development of hypothyroidism. GD is associated with hyperthyroidism and elevated anti-TS--receptor antibodies (TSHR-Ab) in about 95% of patients, in addition to elevated TPO-Ab and anti-thyroglobulin antibodies in some patients.

On ultrasound, the thyroid gland in HT is heterogeneous and hypoechoic with asymmetrical enlargement, lobulated margins and an echogenic capsule. In keeping with the natural history of HT, these changes are progressive and in long-standing disease the echogenicity of the gland is similar to that of the strap muscles of the neck. Hypoechogenicity has been shown to correlate with the risk of developing hypothyroidism in euthyroid patients with HT, and with the degree of hypothyroidism in patients with established thyroid dysfunction [173, 174]. Hypoechogenicity may be initially more apparent in the ventral aspect of the thyroid gland (Image **55**) and eventually involves the whole gland in long-standing disease [11]. While relatively specific for HT, hypoechogenicity of the thyroid gland may be seen in up to two-thirds of morbidly obese euthyroid patients with negative thyroid autoantibodies [175].

Micronodulation, defined as multiple solid, hypoechoic, subcentimetric (1-7 mm) thyroid nodules surrounded by an echogenic rim, is another highly specific feature of HT giving the thyroid gland a 'Swiss cheese' appearance (Image **60**). It has a PPV of 95% for the diagnosis of HT [176]. Other common ultrasound features of HT [11] include distortion of the thyroid architecture and the development of bright fibrous bands (Image **54**) giving the gland a 'honeycomb' like appearance (Image **57**) with separation of thyroid tissue into nodule-like structures termed 'pseudonodules' that may be confused with discrete thyroid nodules. In addition, HT is associated with the development of regenerative hyperechoic nodules known as 'white knights' that may be innumerable giving the gland a 'bag of marbles' appearance (Images **58** and **59**), as well as extra-nodular and intra-nodular macro- and micro-calcifications (Image **61**), and cervical lymphadenopathy most prominent in the central compartment of the neck although the lateral nodes may also be affected.

Central nodes in HT are usually plump, hypoechoic and may have a round shape without a discernible fatty hilum. Despite their concerning ultrasound features, these nodes are often reactive and display little change with serial ultrasound monitoring, however FNA biopsy should be considered if malignancy is suspected. Thyroid gland colour Doppler changes in HT are variable (Image **56**), and may be normal, increased or decreased. Atrophic thyroiditis is characterised on ultrasound by a shrunken, heterogeneous and predominantly hypoechoic thyroid gland (Image **62**), often with micronodulation similar to that seen in HT [11].

Thyroid lymphoma is a rare tumour that occurs almost exclusively in patients with HT. It presents clinically as a rapidly enlarging thyroid mass that on ultrasound appears hypoechoic with increased sound wave transmission posterior to the tumour. FNA biopsy of suspected thyroid lesions with flow cytometry is usually diagnostic.

The ultrasound features of GD are less striking than those of HT. The thyroid gland appears slightly heterogeneous (Image **50**), and is often diffusely enlarged. Hypoechogenicity of the thyroid parenchyma is much less common than in HT, but if present, it may be associated with lower remission rates of hyperthyroidism in response to anti-thyroid medications [177]. Increased Doppler flow is present during the active phase of the disease and may be very intense giving rise to the term 'thyroid inferno' (Image **49**). Increased vascularity of the thyroid may have a prognostic value as to the likelihood of relapse after discontinuation of anti-thyroid medications [178, 179] (Image **51**). There is a 3-fold increase in the prevalence of palpable thyroid nodules in patients with GD compared to the general population, and although up to 17% of palpable nodules may harbour malignancy [180], the overall risk of thyroid cancer in GD is estimated to be low at less than 2% [181]. The approach to thyroid nodule management in GD is similar to that in euthyroid patients, with the exception that a thyroid radioiodine uptake scan may provide useful information about the nodule's risk of malignancy. FNA biopsy should be considered for sonographically suspicious thyroid nodules with poor uptake on thyroid nuclear scan (Image **52**).

Subacute (De Quervain's) thyroiditis is a non-autoimmune condition, possibly of viral origin, that presents with hyperthyroidism and an enlarged, tender thyroid gland with raised erythrocyte sedimentation rate (ESR). It is often preceded by an upper respiratory tract infection and thyroid autoantibodies are not elevated. Thyroid ultrasound examination in subacute thyroiditis is characterised by patchy hypoechoic areas with reduced colour Doppler flow. Incidental thyroid nodules are often seen on ultrasound as they are relatively common in middle-aged women, in whom subacute thyroiditis occurs most frequently. In contrast, silent thyroiditis is an autoimmune condition that presents with mild hyperthyroidism in the absence of thyroid pain or tenderness and a normal ESR. Thyroid scintigraphy shows little or no uptake and up to 50% of patients have elevated TPO-Ab. Post-partum thyroiditis is a variant of silent thyroiditis that occurs in women within 1-year of childbirth. In patients with silent thyroiditis, the thyroid gland is slightly hypoechoic on ultrasound and may display some of the other features of HT as described above.

AIH occurs in up to 20% of patients receiving amiodarone, which has a high iodine content (approximately 40% of its molecular weight). There are two types of AIH: Type 1 presents with a diffuse goitre and normal or increased uptake on thyroid nuclear scan similar to that of Graves' disease. The more common type 2 AIH is destructive thyroiditis with a small goitre and reduced or absent uptake on thyroid nuclear scan. Colour Doppler of the thyroid is an important tool in distinguishing between the two types of AIH, as Doppler flow is typically increased in type 1 and normal or absent in type 2 AIH. Nevertheless, some patients have mixed features of the two AIH types.

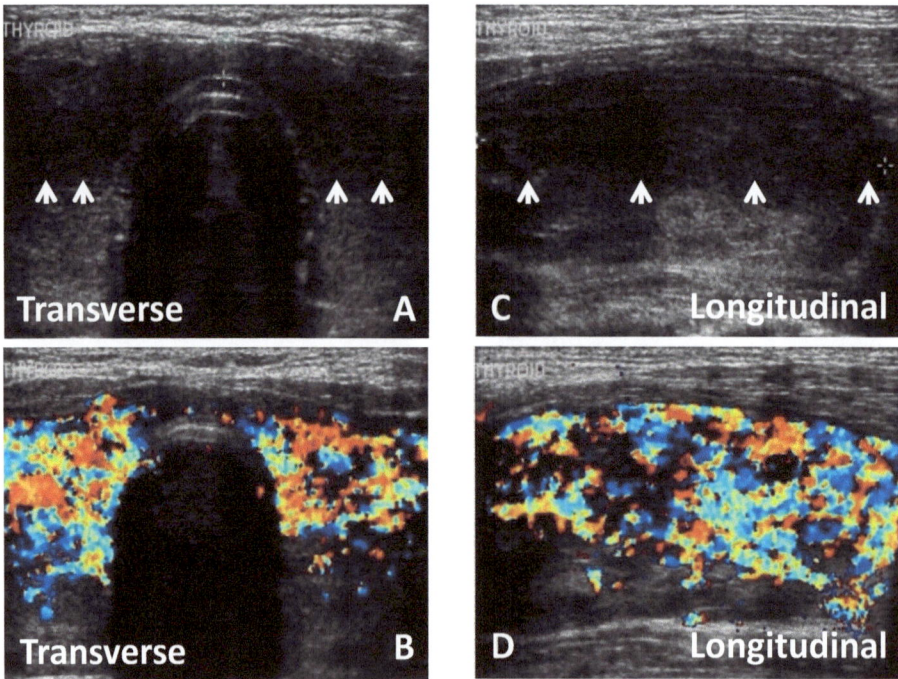

Image (49). Active phase of Graves' hyperthyroidism, transverse and longitudinal planes. There is symmetrical enlargement of the thyroid gland [total volume > 40 cc] and the ventral aspect of the gland is hypoechoic relative to the posterior zone (arrows, A & C). On Doppler flow imaging [B, D], there is an intense increase in vascularity 'thyroid inferno' especially at the ventral aspect of the gland corresponding to the hypoechoic regions in images A and C.

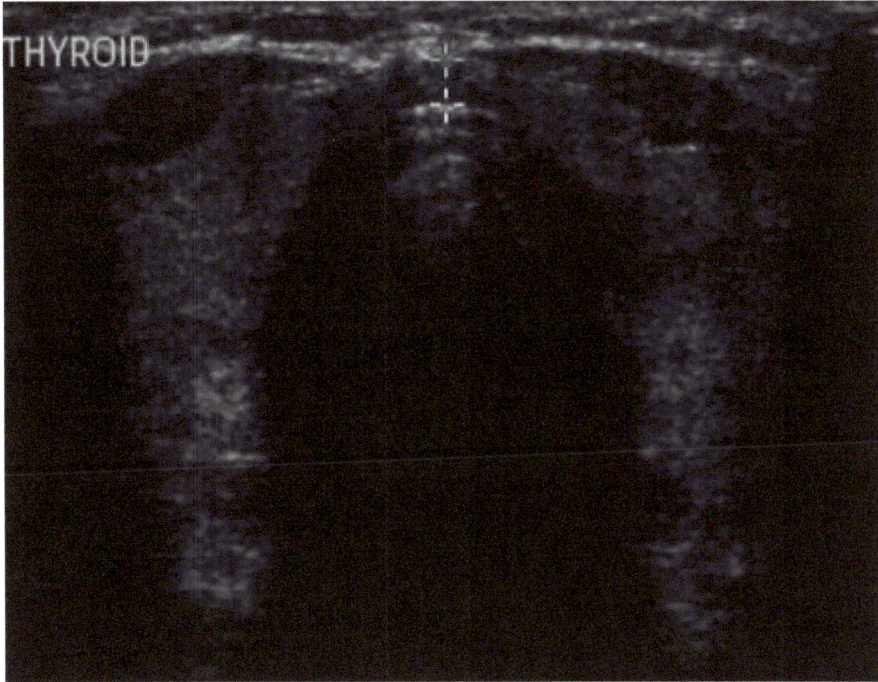

Image (50). Graves' hyperthyroidism with increased heterogeneity of the thyroid gland in B-mode ultrasound imaging. The thyroid gland volume [12 cc] is within normal limits. This is a favourable factor associated with an increased rate of disease remission in response to anti-thyroid medications.

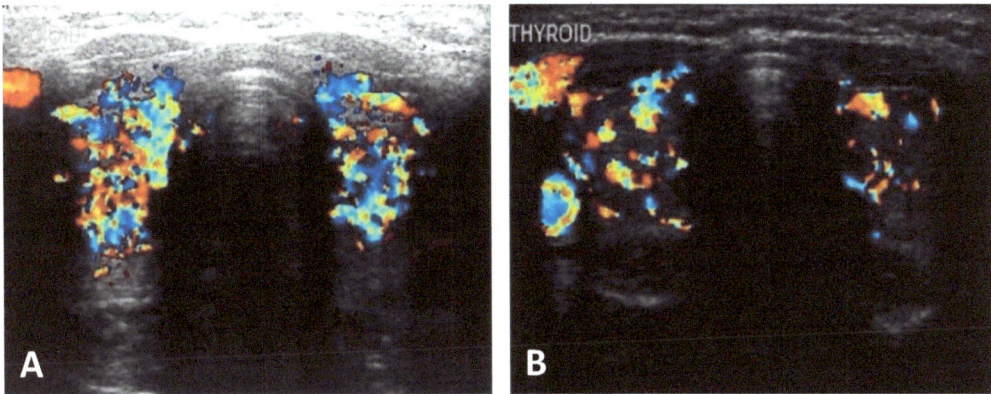

Image (51). Graves' hyperthyroidism before (A) and after (B) treatment with anti-thyroid medications. Note the intense increase in Doppler flow throughout the thyroid gland before treatment (A), while post-treatment Doppler flow (B) is less intense, patchy, and coincides with a reduction in serum thyroid hormone levels.

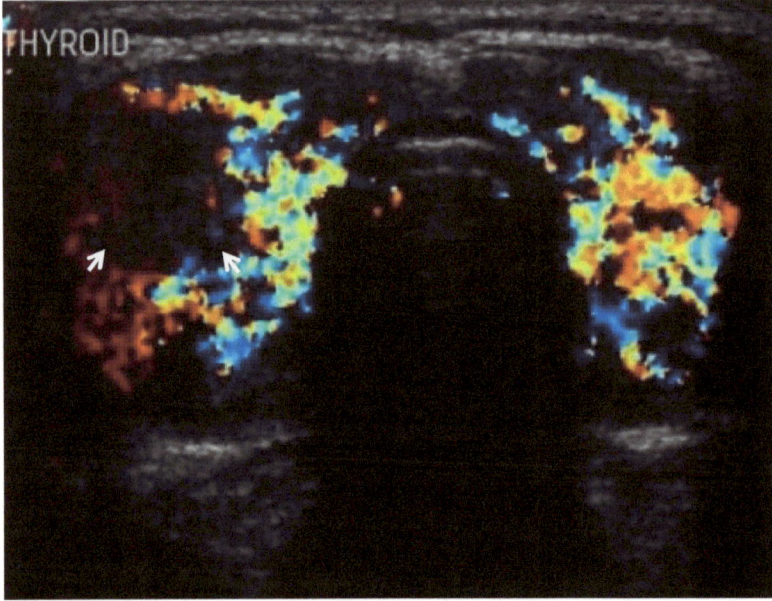

Image (52). Graves' hyperthyroidism with a 2 cm right thyroid isoechoic nodule that was reported 'cold' on thyroid scintigraphy. Note the intense increase in thyroid gland vascularity with sparing of the right thyroid nodule (arrows). FNA biopsy of this nodule is indicated to exclude malignancy.

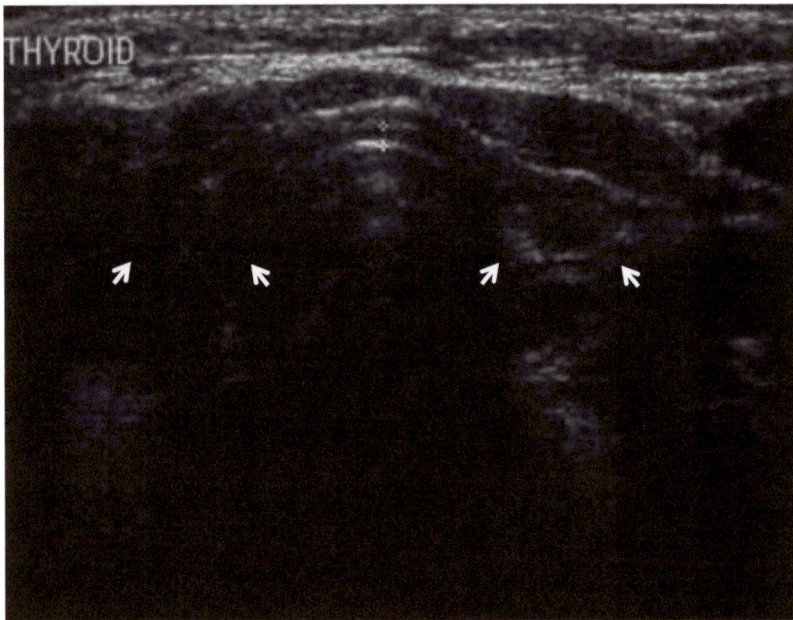

Image (53). Thyroid gland atrophy years post-radioactive iodine ablation for Graves' hyperthyroidism. The gland is heterogeneous with ill-defined margins. The arrows delineate the posterior borders of the gland.

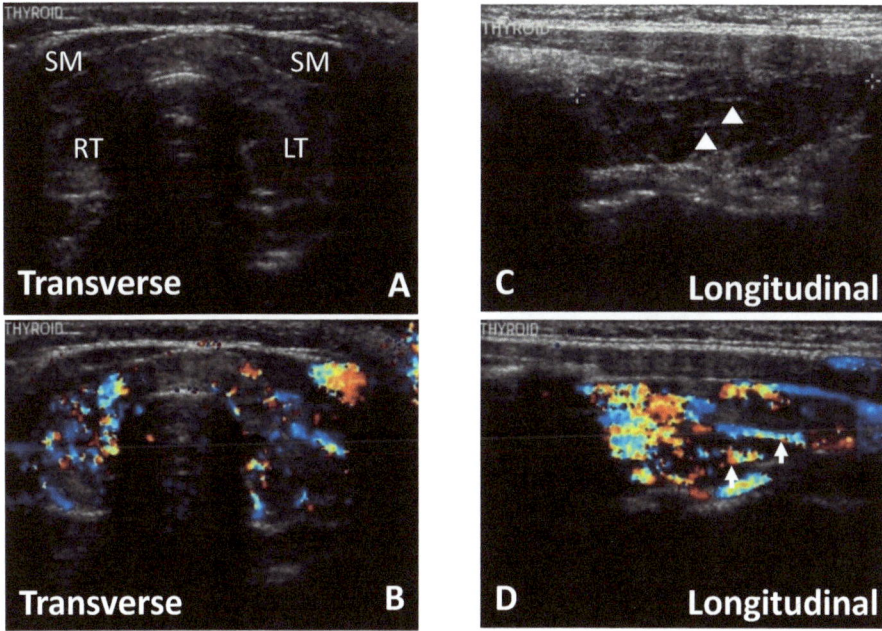

Image (54). Hashimoto's thyroiditis, transverse and longitudinal planes. The thyroid gland is heterogeneous and asymmetrical with a slightly larger left lobe (A). The echogenic fibrous bands are best appreciated in the longitudinal view (arrowheads, C). There is moderate intensity heterogeneous hypervascularity of the thyroid gland [B & D], resembling 'fire stripes' [arrows; D] distributed in the direction of the avascular fibrous bands. SM - strap muscles of the neck, LT – left thyroid lobe, RT – right thyroid lobe.

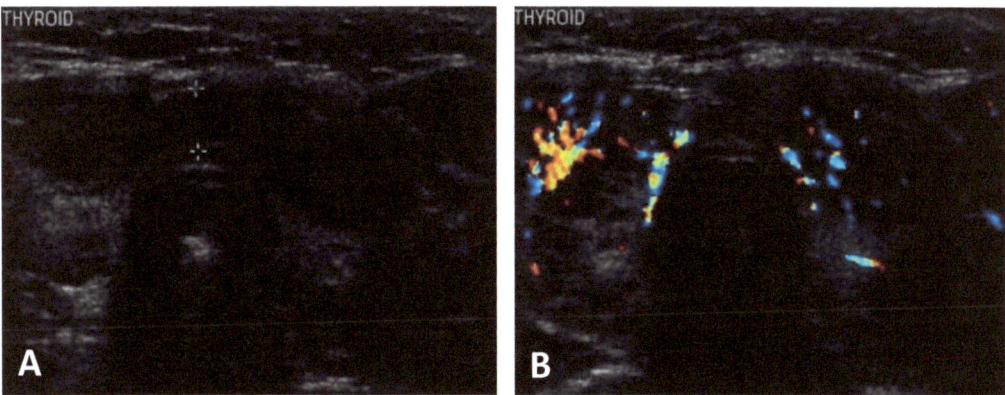

Image (55). Hashimoto's thyroiditis, transverse plane, displaying thyroid gland heterogeneity, hypoechogenicity (A) and patchy increase in vascularity (B) affecting preferentially the ventrum of the thyroid gland. Note mildly increased isthmus width at 0.6 cm.

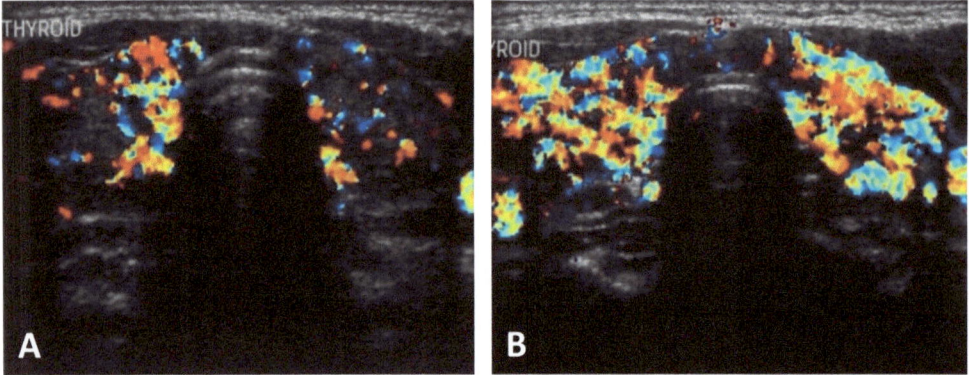

Image (56). Hashimoto's thyroiditis, transverse plane, displaying varying degrees of thyroid gland hypervascularity in different patients. (A) depicts moderate intensity heterogeneous increase in Doppler flow, whereas (B) shows intense hypervascularity similar to that of active Graves' disease.

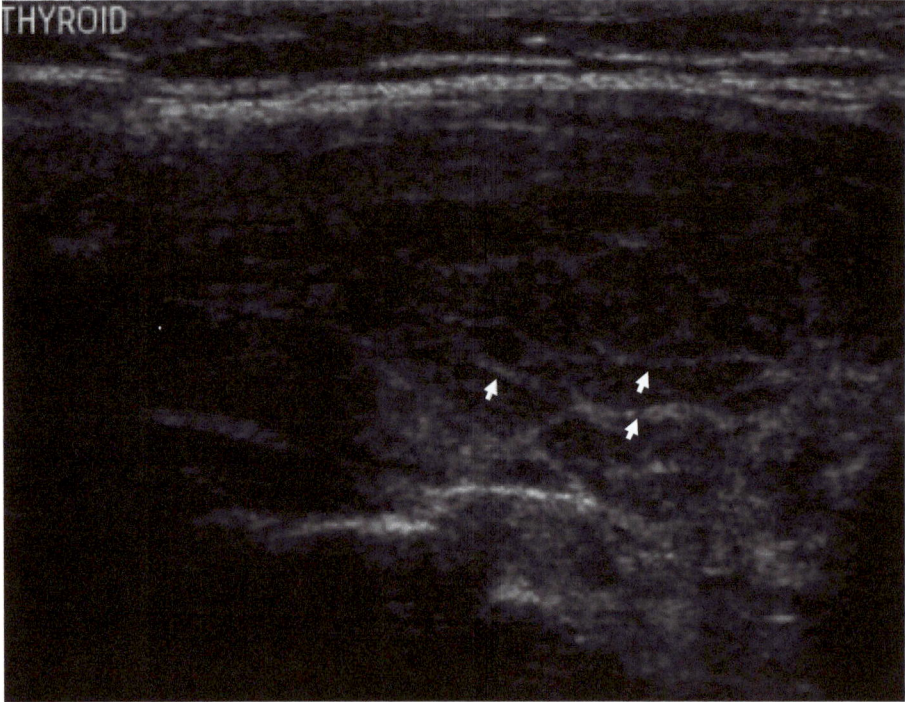

Image (57). Left thyroid lobe, longitudinal plane, in a patient with Hashimoto's thyroiditis. The thyroid parenchyma is heterogeneous and hypoechoic, with multiple echogenic fibrous bands [arrows] aligned predominantly along the longitudinal axis of the thyroid gland creating a 'honeycomb' pattern that may give rise to nodule-like structures termed 'pseudonodules'.

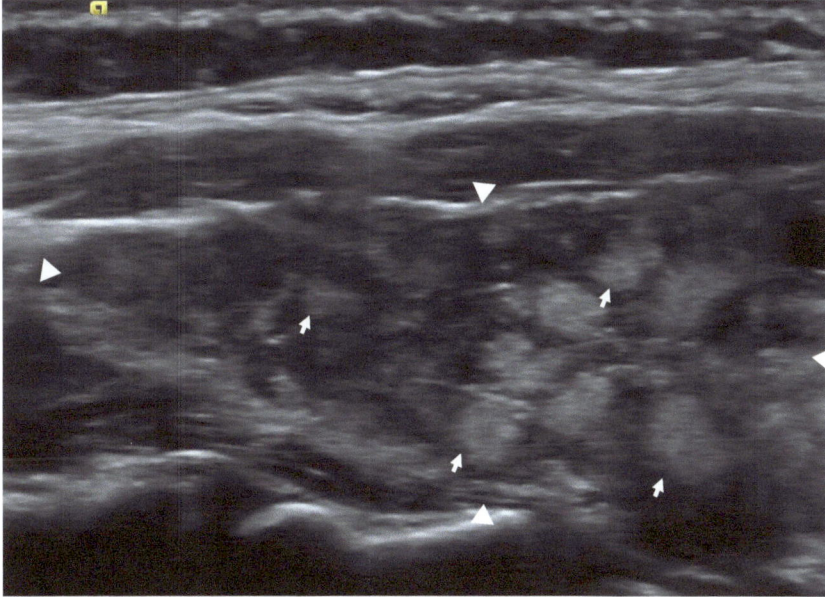

Image (58). Left thyroid lobe, longitudinal plane, displaying multiple hyperechoic nodules (arrows) in a patient with Hashimoto's thyroiditis giving the thyroid gland the appearance of a 'bag of marbles'. These regenerative thyroid nodules are known as 'white knights' and have a low suspicion for malignancy (see text for further details and references).

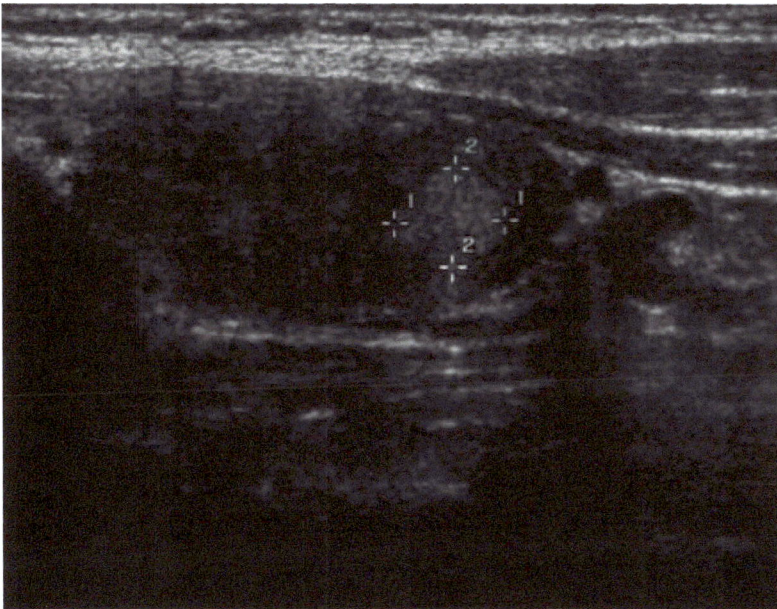

Image (59). Hashimoto's thyroiditis with a hyperechoic right inferior thyroid nodule, likely representing a regenerative nodule 'white knight' with a low suspicion of malignancy.

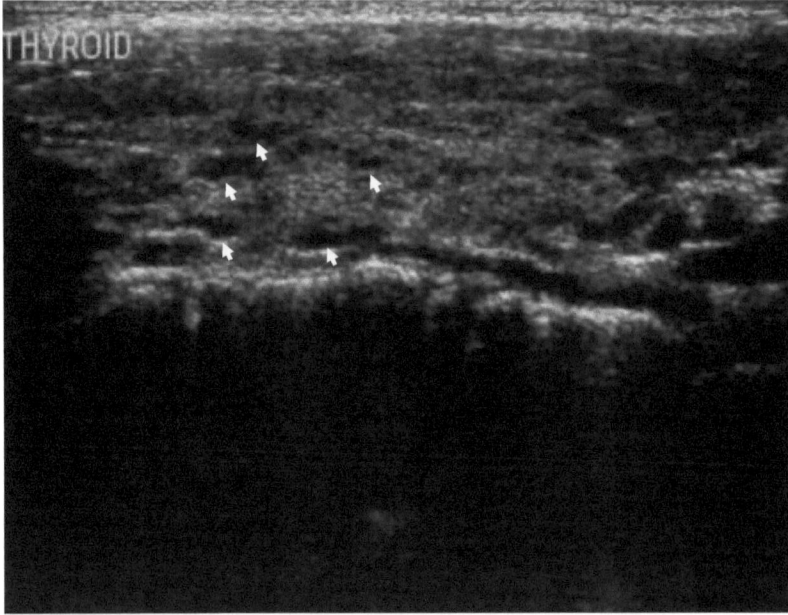

Image (60). Right thyroid lobe, longitudinal plane, in Hashimoto's thyroiditis. Note multiple tiny hypoechoic solid subcentimetric nodules (arrows). Termed 'micronodulation', this feature is highly specific for Hashimoto's thyroiditis.

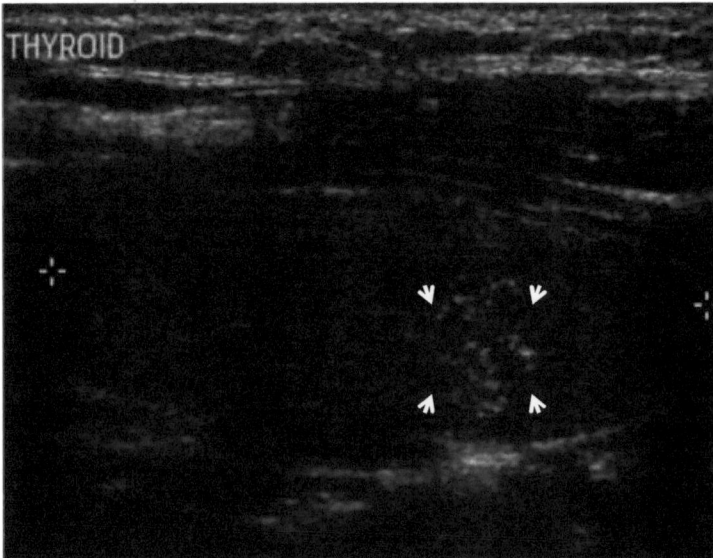

Image (61). Hashimoto's thyroiditis, longitudinal plane, displaying a focus of intense microcalcification (arrows). While a discrete nodule was not apparent, in the presence of distorted thyroid architecture FNA biopsy of the suspicious region is warranted to exclude malignancy.

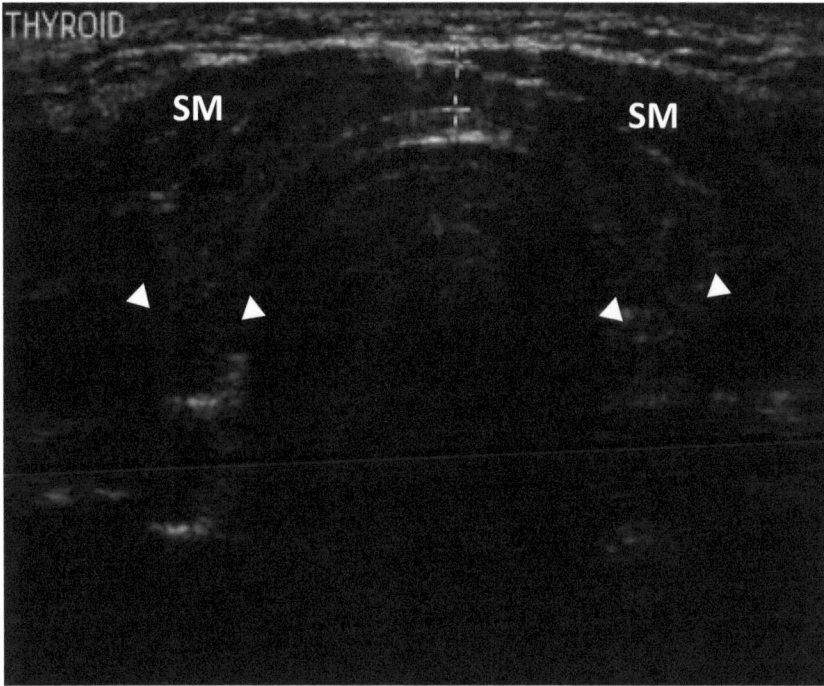

Image (62). Autoimmune 'atrophic' thyroiditis, transverse plane, displaying a hypoechoic and shrunken thyroid gland of similar echogenicity to the strap muscles of the neck [SM].

CHAPTER 10

Ultrasound of Parathyroid Glands

Abstract: When considering surgery for the treatment of primary hyperparathyroidism, accurate pre-operative localisation of the hyperfunctioning parathyroid adenoma is associated with successful resection of the adenoma and correction of hypercalcaemia using minimally invasive parathyroid surgery. Hyperparathyroidism is most commonly caused by a single parathyroid adenoma, while multiple gland hyperplasia is less common and parathyroid carcinoma is rarely encountered. Neck ultrasound is an excellent tool for the localisation of a single parathyroid adenoma and allows examination of the thyroid gland for thyroid nodules which are seen in up to 40% of patients with hyperparathyroidism. The presence of thyroid nodules requires pre-operative evaluation and exclusion of thyroid malignancy and may change the surgical approach. Parathyroid scintigraphy is complementary to ultrasound with the added advantage of identifying an ectopic parathyroid adenoma outside the field of ultrasound imaging. Parathyroid ultrasound and scintigraphy are both less sensitive for the detection of multiple parathyroid gland hyperplasia. Parathyroid gland fine needle aspiration biopsy and measurement of parathyroid hormone in the needle washout confirms the diagnosis when parathyroid imaging is inconclusive.

Keywords: Cervical lymphadenopathy, Colour Doppler study, Ectopic, Feeding artery, Fine needle aspiration, Neck ultrasound, Parathyroid adenoma, Parathyroid hyperplasia, Parathyroid carcinoma, Parathyroid lipoadenoma, Parathyroid nuclear scan, Primary hyperparathyroidism, Parathyroid hormone, Parathyromatosis, Parathyroid exploration, Parathyroidectomy, Thyroid nodule.

Primary hyperparathyroidism may be due to a single parathyroid adenoma (85% of cases), multiple gland hyperplasia or multiple adenomas (15%), and rarely, a carcinoma [182]. While most people have four parathyroid glands, up to 20% have fewer or more than four glands [183], and 1-3% of glands are ectopic [184, 185]. As discussed in the anatomy section, the parathyroid glands may be located anywhere from the lower mandible to the pericardium with a greater variability in the position of the inferior than the superior glands. Recent advances in parathyroid imaging allow accurate pre-operative localization of a single parathyroid adenoma and the use of minimally invasive surgery to excise these glands. However, parathyroid imaging is less helpful and is often negative in multiglandular disease [186 - 188].

Normal parathyroid glands measure 5 mm or less and may be difficult to visualise with ultrasound [189]. In primary hyperparathyroidism, normal parathyroids may be even smaller due to suppression of their function. Pre-operative neck ultrasonography provides structural information about the parathyroids and identifies co-existant thyroid nodules in up to 40% of patients with an estimated thyroid malignancy risk of 2-6% [190 - 192], which may alter the surgical approach to hyperparathyroidism. In contrast, a parathyroid nuclear scan confirms hyperfunction of an enlarged parathyroid gland.

Parathyroid ultrasonography is best performed with a high frequency [12-15 MHz] linear transducer. It is usually carried out at the same time as the neck and thyroid ultrasound. The patient is placed in the same position as for thyroid ultrasonography with the neck extended by placing a pillow behind the shoulders. The area of greatest interest during the examination is located between the two carotid arteries from the clavicles inferiorly to the hyoid bone superiorly. The superior parathyroids are commonly found posterior to the middle third of the thyroid gland and the inferior parathyroids at the inferior border of the thyroid. Ectopic locations for the superior parathyroids include retro-oesophageal space, inferior mediastinum and intra-thyroidal. Ectopic inferior parathyroids may be found in the carotid sheath, anterior mediastinum, intra-thymic or intra-thyroidal [193]. Having the patient turn their head slightly away from the side being examined may expose an ectopic superior parathyroid gland in the trachea-oesophageal groove. In addition, asking the patient to swallow while imaging may identify parathyroid glands located below the clavicular line.

On ultrasound, parathyroid adenomas appear as hypoechoic oval-shaped structures separated from the thyroid gland by the hyperechoic thyroid capsule (Images **63** and **64**). Normal and hyperplastic parathyroid glands are more difficult to visualize on ultrasound due to their smaller size and isoechogenicity relative to the thyroid gland [182]. Colour Doppler can help identify a feeding artery to suspected parathyroid tumours.

The feeding artery may be seen in up to 60% of parathyroid adenomas [194] and resembles a vascular arc at the periphery of the adenoma (Image **65**). Parathyroid glands may be bi-lobed or multi-lobed in up to 5% of cases [184], cystic (Image **66**) or partially cystic in 1-2% and rarely they may appear hyperechoic which is suggestive of a lipid-rich parathyroid lipoadenoma. The rare parathyroid carcinoma is suspected on ultrasound by the presence of a heterogeneous parathyroid gland that is taller-than-wide with ill-defined margins [195].

The distinction between central cervical lymphadenopathy in Hashimoto's thyroiditis and a parathyroid adenoma by ultrasound may not be straightforward.

While the absence of a feeding artery does not exclude a parathyroid adenoma, a fatty hilum with or without central vascularity is consistent with cervical lymphadenopathy.

In primary hyperparathyroidism, the sensitivity of ultrasound for the detection of a solitary parathyroid adenoma is robust at 80% but is much lower in multiglandular disease (35%) and in parathyroid hyperplasia (16%) [196]. Parathyroid scintigraphy has a similar sensitivity for the detection of a single parathyroid adenoma although when combined with ultrasound, the sensitivity increases to 74-95% [188, 197, 198]. Parathyroid scintigraphy has the added advantage of detecting ectopic parathyroid glands situated outside of the ultrasound imaging field. Concordance between neck ultrasound and parathyroid nuclear scans leads to correct surgical localization of a parathyroid adenoma with minimally invasive parathyroid surgery and correction of hypercalcemia in up to 95% of cases [199].

However, even the combination of parathyroid ultrasonography and scintigraphy has a poor sensitivity (30%) for the detection of multiglandular disease and parathyroid hyperplasia, and it is worth noting that up to 30% of patient with concordant imaging for a solitary parathyroid adenoma may have multiglandular disease [200]. For this reason, many surgeons rely on intra-operative PTH monitoring to guide the course of surgery and decide if they need to switch from a selective surgical approach to bilateral parathyroid exploration.

FNA biopsy of a suspected parathyroid gland and measurement of PTH in the needle washout should be considered when neck ultrasonography findings are in disagreement with other imaging modalities such as parathyroid scintigraphy. Elevation of the FNA-PTH above the serum PTH is diagnostic of a parathyroid adenoma [191]. Seeding of parathyroid cells along the needle tract, known as parathyromatosis, is a rare complication of FNA biopsy of the parathyroid gland.

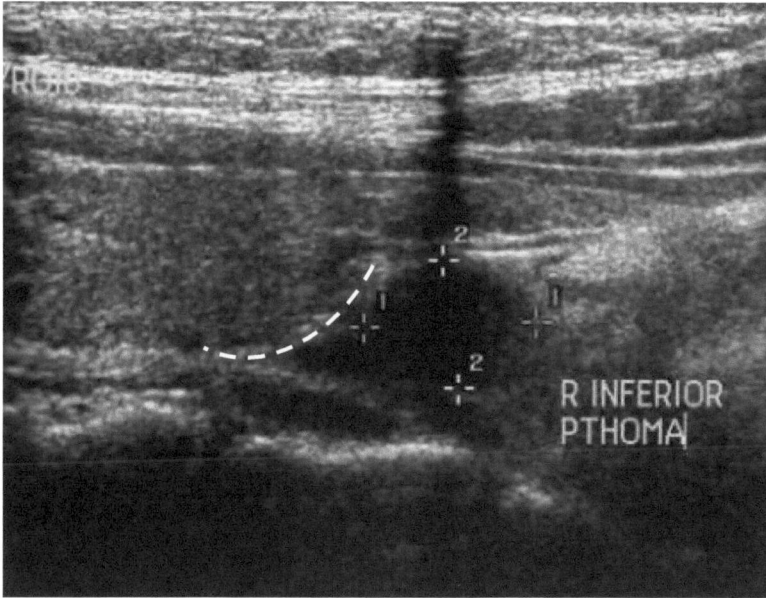

Image (63). Right thyroid longitudinal plane demonstrating a right inferior parathyroid adenoma measuring 1.1 x 0.8 cm in a patient with hypercalcaemia and elevated plasma parathyroid hormone levels. Note the ill-defined, hypoechoic, round structure separated from the thyroid parenchyma by the thyroid capsule (dashed line). A parathyroid nuclear scan confirmed the presence of a right inferior parathyroid adenoma.

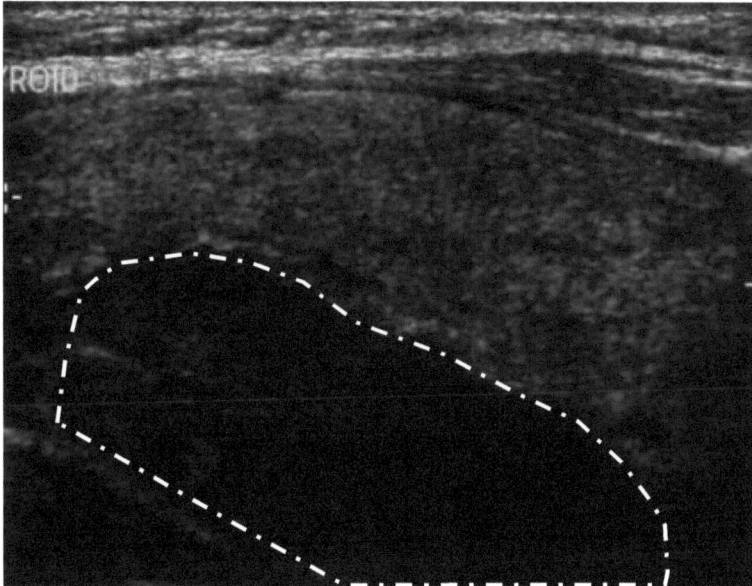

Image (64). Left thyroid longitudinal plane demonstrating a large left parathyroid adenoma measuring 4.4 x 1.8 cm. The adenoma is hypoechoic, lies posteriorly to the left lobe of the thyroid. A distinct margin between the thyroid gland and the parathyroid adenoma may not always be appreciated, as in this case.

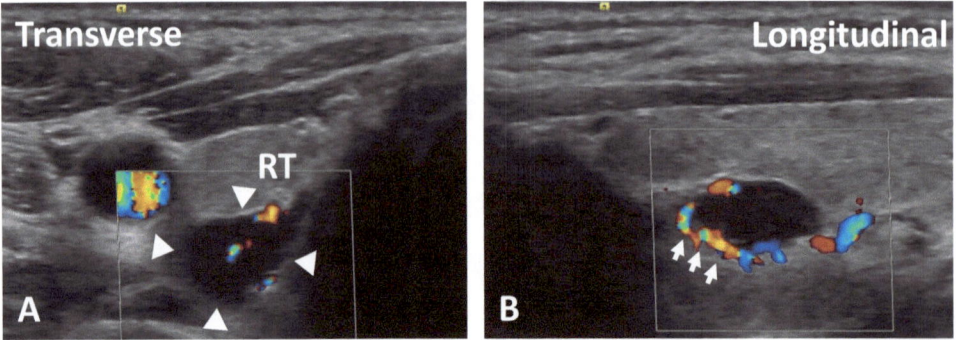

Image (65). Right upper parathyroid adenoma measuring 1.1 cm, transverse (A) and longitudinal (B) planes. Note hypoechoic parathyroid adenoma (arrowheads, A) situated at the posterior border of the right (RT) thyroid lobe. A feeding artery that resembles a vascular arc can be seen in the longitudinal view (arrows, B).

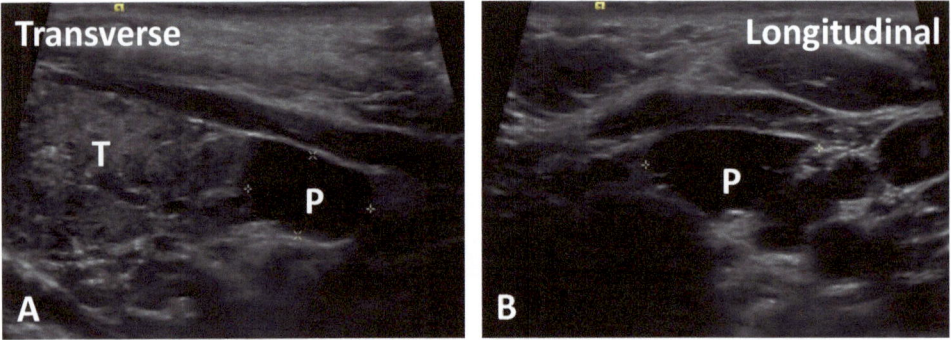

Image (66). Left inferior parathyroid cyst (P), longitudinal (A) and transverse (B) planes, in a patient with normal plasma calcium and elevated plasma parathyroid hormone. The cyst is hypoechoic with posterior enhancement. Note heterogeneous thyroid gland (T) in keeping with a history of Hashimoto's thyroiditis. FNA biopsy of the cyst revealed a very high parathyroid hormone from the needle washout (FNA-PTH 530 pmol/L) thereby confirming the diagnosis, although the specimen was acellular. In normocalcaemic hyperparathyroidism, surgical excision of the parathyroid adenoma may be considered in patients with skeletal or renal manifestations of hyperparathyroidism.

CHAPTER 11

Percutaneous Ethanol Injection

Abstract: Percutaneous ethanol injection post-fluid aspiration of pure thyroid cysts and predominantly cystic thyroid nodules is highly effective in preventing fluid re-accumulation. The procedure is simple, safe and is performed in the outpatient clinic under ultrasound guidance. A coordinated approach between the physician and an experienced assistant who controls fluid aspiration and alcohol injection is essential. Before ablation is undertaken, FNA biopsy of the solid component is essential to exclude malignancy. Any suspicious thyroid nodules should also be biopsied. Alcohol leakage is an uncommon but serious complication of percutaneous ethanol injection and may lead to voice changes due to demyelination of the recurrent laryngeal nerve. The trans-isthmic approach may be associated with a lower risk of ethanol leakage. Percutaneous ethanol injection is also effective for the ablation of metastatic cervical lymph nodes in thyroid cancer patients and may avoid the need for re-operation. However, ethanol ablation is not the first option in hyperfunctioning thyroid nodules and parathyroid adenomas due to poor response rates.

Keywords: cystic, thyroid nodule, percutaneous, ethanol, ablation, thyroid nodule volume, aspiration, two-way valve, trans-isthmic, ethanol leakage, nerve demyelination, proteinaceous, parathyroid adenoma, malignant cervical nodes, berry picking.

Ablation of cystic thyroid nodules using Percutaneous Ethanol Injection (PEI) was first reported by Rozman *et al.* [201, 202]. PEI is indicated for large predominantly cystic nodules that may or may not be associated with neck compressive symptoms. The procedure is safe, effective and leads to durable nodule volume reductions exceeding 75% after an average of two treatments, although the success rates are lower in predominantly cystic vascular nodules compared with purely cystic nodules [44]. Potential complications include local pain, dysphonia, Horner's syndrome, infection, flushing and dizziness [44, 203 - 205]. In contrast to PEI, thyroid cyst aspiration alone has a high recurrence rate and fluid re-accumulation is seen in up to 90% of nodules [204].

A baseline ultrasound scan of the thyroid gland allows estimation of the cystic content of the nodule, whether intranodular septations are present, and the risk of

Samer El-Kaissi & Jack R Wall

malignancy of the solid component of the nodule is assessed. In addition, the thyroid ultrasound often identifies other nodules and determines their suspicion of malignancy. Our approach is to perform an initial cyst aspiration and FNA biopsy of the solid component and any suspicious nodules. If cytology is reported as benign, the patient is scheduled for repeat ultrasound after 1-month to assess fluid reaccumulation and to perform PEI if required.

On the day of the procedure, the benefits and potential risks of PEI are explained to the patient and an informed consent is obtained. The patient is positioned and prepared as described in the FNA biopsy section above. Using a flexible tube, a 1.5" long needle (22-25G), is attached to one end of the tube and a two-way valve is attached to the other end. Two syringes are attached to the two-way valve, an empty syringe for aspiration of cyst contents and the other syringe containing 95% sterile ethanol for injection. This avoids the need for a second puncture that may increase the risk of extravasation of the ethanol into surrounding tissues [202] The size of the aspiration syringe depends on the estimated volume of the cyst.

After localization of the cystic thyroid nodule to be ablated with ethanol, the needle is introduced into the cyst under ultrasound guidance and contents of the cyst are aspirated, after which the assistant switches the two-way valve and begins PEI slowly. The volume of ethanol that is injected is approximately half of the volume of aspirated cyst fluid, to a maximum of 20 ml. A parallel needle path is preferred as it allows visualization of the whole needle throughout the procedure. It is important to keep the bevel of the needle in view at the centre of the cystic nodule at all times and if the bevel touches the wall of the nodule, the procedure is aborted and re-scheduled after 1-month [202]. Alcohol injection should also be aborted if any resistance is encountered. This procedure requires great coordination between the physician who is holding the ultrasound probe and keeping the bevel of the needle in view throughout the procedure, and the assistant controlling fluid aspiration and ethanol injection.

The trans-isthmic approach is an alternative PEI method that has the advantages of reduced needle tip movement and potentially lower rates of ethanol leakage. Using this technique, a 14-18 G needle is inserted *via* the isthmus into the nodule to be ablated. After thyroid nodule fluid aspiration and saline irrigation of the nodule to remove debris, ethanol is injected and retained in the nodule for 2 minutes followed by complete removal of the ethanol [44].

Cysts that contain highly proteinaceous fluid preventing adequate aspiration can be injected with a small amount of ethanol, approximately 10% of the estimated cyst volume. Within 2-weeks, the proteinaceous fluid undergoes liquefaction thereby allowing aspiration of cyst contents and performance of PEI [206].

Apart from cystic thyroid nodules, PEI has been described for hyperfunctioning thyroid nodules [207], parathyroid adenomas [208] and metastatic CLN [209 - 211]. Despite the high short-term success rates of PEI of autonomous thyroid nodules [212], recurrence is common [205] and PEI is currently not recommended for toxic nodules unless other treatment modalities are not available. Similarly, only one-third of patients with primary hyperparathyroidism remains hypocalcaemic post-PEI of a parathyroid adenoma suggesting that PEI should be reserved for inoperable parathyroid disease [213]. Furthermore, Thyroid adenomas often lack a thick capsule thereby increasing the risk of ethanol spillage into surrounding tissues which may result in demyelination of the recurrent and/or superior laryngeal nerves [214].

PEI of malignant CLNs is highly effective and a retrospective study of 109 metastatic PTC CLNs by Heilo *et al.* reported a 93% response rate to ultrasound-guided PEI (0.1-1.0 ml) with 84% of the CLNs showing a complete response over a mean follow-up period of 38-months [209]. Colour Doppler imaging was used to ensure the loss of CLN vascularization after PEI. The authors suggest that up to five malignant CLN can be treated and that PEI could replace 'berry-picking' in post-operative PTC patients with lymph node metastases. However, long-term prognostic data is still lacking for this procedure.

REFERENCES

[1]   Coltrera MD. Ultrasound physics in a nutshell. Otolaryngologic clinics of North America 2010; 43(6): 1149-59. v. Epub 2010/11/04
        [http://dx.doi.org/10.1016/j.otc.2010.08.004]

[2]   Uppal T. Tissue harmonic imaging. Australas J Ultrasound Med 2010; 13(2): 29-31.
        [http://dx.doi.org/10.1002/j.2205-0140.2010.tb00155.x]

[3]   Levine RA. Something old and something new: a brief history of thyroid ultrasound technology. Endocr Pract 2004; 10(3): 227-33.
        [http://dx.doi.org/10.4158/EP.10.3.227]

[4]   Uppal T, Mogra R. RBC motion and the basis of ultrasound Doppler instrumentation. Australas J Ultrasound Med 2010; 13(1): 32-4.
        [http://dx.doi.org/10.1002/j.2205-0140.2010.tb00216.x]

[5]   J. Shrik. Ultrasound physics. Critical care clinics 2014; 30(1): 1-24. v. Epub 2013/12/04

[6]   Klem C. Head and neck anatomy and ultrasound correlation Otolaryngologic clinics of North America 2010; 43(6): 1161-9. v. Epub 2010/11/04

[7]   Policeni BA, Smoker WR, Reede DL. Anatomy and embryology of the thyroid and parathyroid glands. Semin Ultrasound CT MR 2012; 33(2): 104-14.
        [http://dx.doi.org/10.1053/j.sult.2011.12.005]

[8]   Morris LF, Ragavendra N, Yeh MW. Evidence-based assessment of the role of ultrasonography in the management of benign thyroid nodules. World J Surg 2008; 32(7): 1253-63.
        [http://dx.doi.org/10.1007/s00268-008-9494-z]

[9]   Guth S, Theune U, Aberle J, Galach A, Bamberger CM. Very high prevalence of thyroid nodules detected by high frequency (13 MHz) ultrasound examination. Eur J Clin Invest 2009; 39(8): 699-706.
        [http://dx.doi.org/10.1111/j.1365-2362.2009.02162.x]

[10]   Hegedus L, Perrild H, Poulsen LR, *et al.* The determination of thyroid volume by ultrasound and its relationship to body weight, age, and sex in normal subjects. J Clin Endocrinol Metab 1983; 56(2): 260-3.
        [http://dx.doi.org/10.1210/jcem-56-2-260]

[11]   Sholosh B, Borhani AA. Thyroid ultrasound part 1: technique and diffuse disease. Radiol Clin North Am 2011; 49(3): 391-416.
        [http://dx.doi.org/10.1016/j.rcl.2011.02.002]

[12]   Ota H, Amino N, Morita S, *et al.* Quantitative measurement of thyroid blood flow for differentiation of painless thyroiditis from Graves' disease. Clin Endocrinol (Oxf) 2007; 67(1): 41-5.
        [http://dx.doi.org/10.1111/j.1365-2265.2007.02832.x]

[13]   Castagnone D, Rivolta R, Rescalli S, Baldini MI, Tozzi R, Cantalamessa L. Color Doppler sonography in Graves' disease: value in assessing activity of disease and predicting outcome. AJR Am J Roentgenol 1996; 166(1): 203-7.
        [http://dx.doi.org/10.2214/ajr.166.1.8571877]

[14]   Saleh A, Cohnen M, Furst G, Godehardt E, Modder U, Feldkamp J. Differential diagnosis of hyperthyroidism: Doppler sonographic quantification of thyroid blood flow distinguishes between Graves' disease and diffuse toxic goiter. Exp Clin Endocrinol Diabetes 2002; 110(1): 32-6.
        [http://dx.doi.org/10.1055/s-2002-19992]

[15]   Bartolotta TV, Midiri M, Galia M, *et al.* Qualitative and quantitative evaluation of solitary thyroid nodules with contrast-enhanced ultrasound: initial results. Eur Radiol 2006; 16(10): 2234-41.
        [http://dx.doi.org/10.1007/s00330-006-0229-y]

[16] Zenk J, Bozzato A, Hornung J, *et al.* Neck lymph nodes: prediction by computer-assisted contrast medium analysis? Ultrasound Med Biol 2007; 33(2): 246-53.
[http://dx.doi.org/10.1016/j.ultrasmedbio.2006.08.005]

[17] Russ G, Bonnema SJ, Erdogan MF, Durante C, Ngu R, Leenhardt L. European Thyroid Association Guidelines for Ultrasound Malignancy Risk Stratification of Thyroid Nodules in Adults: The EU-TIRADS. Eur Thyroid J 2017; 6: 225-37.
[http://dx.doi.org/10.1159/000478927]

[18] Tunbridge WM, Evered DC, Hall R, *et al.* The spectrum of thyroid disease in a community: the Whickham survey. Clin Endocrinol (Oxf) 1977; 7(6): 481-93.
[http://dx.doi.org/10.1111/j.1365-2265.1977.tb01340.x]

[19] Tan GH, Gharib H. Thyroid incidentalomas: management approaches to nonpalpable nodules discovered incidentally on thyroid imaging. Ann Intern Med 1997; 126(3): 226-31.
[http://dx.doi.org/10.7326/0003-4819-126-3-199702010-00009]

[20] Mortensen JD, Woolner LB, Bennett WA. Gross and microscopic findings in clinically normal thyroid glands. J Clin Endocrinol Metab 1955; 15(10): 1270-80.
[http://dx.doi.org/10.1210/jcem-15-10-1270]

[21] Hegedus L. Clinical practice. The thyroid nodule. N Engl J Med 2004; 351(17): 1764-71.
[http://dx.doi.org/10.1056/NEJMcp031436]

[22] Mandel SJ. Diagnostic use of ultrasonography in patients with nodular thyroid disease. Endocr Pract 2004; 10(3): 246-52.
[http://dx.doi.org/10.4158/EP.10.3.246]

[23] Papini E, Guglielmi R, Bianchini A, *et al.* Risk of malignancy in nonpalpable thyroid nodules: predictive value of ultrasound and color-Doppler features. J Clin Endocrinol Metab 2002; 87(5): 1941-6.
[http://dx.doi.org/10.1210/jcem.87.5.8504]

[24] McCall A, Jarosz H, Lawrence AM, Paloyan E. The incidence of thyroid carcinoma in solitary cold nodules and in multinodular goiters. Surgery 1986; 100(6): 1128-32.

[25] Frates MC, Benson CB, Charboneau JW, *et al.* Management of thyroid nodules detected at US: Society of Radiologists in Ultrasound consensus conference statement. Radiology 2005; 237(3): 794-800.
[http://dx.doi.org/10.1148/radiol.2373050220]

[26] Frates MC, Benson CB, Doubilet PM, *et al.* Prevalence and distribution of carcinoma in patients with solitary and multiple thyroid nodules on sonography. J Clin Endocrinol Metab 2006; 91(9): 3411-7.
[http://dx.doi.org/10.1210/jc.2006-0690]

[27] Sherman SI. Thyroid carcinoma. Lancet 2003; 361(9356): 501-11.
[http://dx.doi.org/10.1016/S0140-6736(03)12488-9]

[28] Lee MJ, Kim EK, Kwak JY, Kim MJ. Partially cystic thyroid nodules on ultrasound: probability of malignancy and sonographic differentiation. Thyroid 2009; 19(4): 341-6.
[http://dx.doi.org/10.1089/thy.2008.0250]

[29] Chan BK, Desser TS, McDougall IR, Weigel RJ, Jeffrey RB Jr. Common and uncommon sonographic features of papillary thyroid carcinoma. J Ultrasound Med 2003; 22(10): 1083-90.
[http://dx.doi.org/10.7863/jum.2003.22.10.1083]

[30] Watters DA, Ahuja AT, Evans RM, *et al.* Role of ultrasound in the management of thyroid nodules. Am J Surg 1992; 164(6): 654-7.
[http://dx.doi.org/10.1016/S0002-9610(05)80728-7]

[31] Machens A, Holzhausen HJ, Dralle H. The prognostic value of primary tumor size in papillary and follicular thyroid carcinoma. Cancer 2005; 103(11): 2269-73.

[http://dx.doi.org/10.1002/cncr.21055]

[32]   Kangelaris GT, Kim TB, Orloff LA. Role of ultrasound in thyroid disorders. Otolaryngol Clin North Am 2010; 43(6): 1209-27. [vi.].
[http://dx.doi.org/10.1016/j.otc.2010.08.006]

[33]   Davies L, Welch HG. Current thyroid cancer trends in the United States. JAMA Otolaryngol Head Neck Surg 2014; 140(4): 317-22.
[http://dx.doi.org/10.1001/jamaoto.2014.1]

[34]   Enewold L, Zhu K, Ron E, *et al.* Rising thyroid cancer incidence in the United States by demographic and tumor characteristics, 1980-2005. Cancer Epidemiol Biomarkers Prev 2009; 18(3): 784-91.
[http://dx.doi.org/10.1158/1055-9965.EPI-08-0960]

[35]   Haugen BR, Alexander EK, Bible KC, *et al.* 2015 American Thyroid Association Management Guidelines for Adult Patients with Thyroid Nodules and Differentiated Thyroid Cancer: The American Thyroid Association Guidelines Task Force on Thyroid Nodules and Differentiated Thyroid Cancer. Thyroid 2016; 26(1): 1-133.
[http://dx.doi.org/10.1089/thy.2015.0020]

[36]   Brito JP, Gionfriddo MR, Al Nofal A, *et al.* The accuracy of thyroid nodule ultrasound to predict thyroid cancer: systematic review and meta-analysis. J Clin Endocrinol Metab 2014; 99(4): 1253-63.
[http://dx.doi.org/10.1210/jc.2013-2928]

[37]   Horvath E, Majlis S, Rossi R, *et al.* An ultrasonogram reporting system for thyroid nodules stratifying cancer risk for clinical management. J Clin Endocrinol Metab 2009; 94(5): 1748-51.
[http://dx.doi.org/10.1210/jc.2008-1724]

[38]   Tae HJ, Lim DJ, Baek KH, *et al.* Diagnostic value of ultrasonography to distinguish between benign and malignant lesions in the management of thyroid nodules. Thyroid 2007; 17(5): 461-6.
[http://dx.doi.org/10.1089/thy.2006.0337]

[39]   Moon WJ, Jung SL, Lee JH, *et al.* Benign and malignant thyroid nodules: US differentiation-multicenter retrospective study. Radiology 2008; 247(3): 762-70.
[http://dx.doi.org/10.1148/radiol.2473070944]

[40]   Gorman B, Charboneau JW, James EM, *et al.* Medullary thyroid carcinoma: role of high-resolution US. Radiology 1987; 162(1 Pt 1): 147-50.
[http://dx.doi.org/10.1148/radiology.162.1.3538147]

[41]   Henrichsen TL, Reading CC. Thyroid ultrasonography. Part 2: nodules. Radiol Clin North Am 2011; 49(3): 417-24.
[http://dx.doi.org/10.1016/j.rcl.2011.02.003]

[42]   Moon HJ, Sung JM, Kim EK, Yoon JH, Youk JH, Kwak JY. Diagnostic performance of gray-scale US and elastography in solid thyroid nodules. Radiology 2012; 262(3): 1002-13.
[http://dx.doi.org/10.1148/radiol.11110839]

[43]   Park YJ, Kim JA, Son EJ, *et al.* Thyroid nodules with macrocalcification: sonographic findings predictive of malignancy. Yonsei Med J 2014; 55(2): 339-44.
[http://dx.doi.org/10.3349/ymj.2014.55.2.339]

[44]   Kim YJ, Baek JH, Ha EJ, *et al.* Cystic *versus* predominantly cystic thyroid nodules: efficacy of ethanol ablation and analysis of related factors. Eur Radiol 2012; 22(7): 1573-8.
[http://dx.doi.org/10.1007/s00330-012-2406-5]

[45]   Holden A. The role of colour and duplex Doppler ultrasound in the assessment of thyroid nodules. Australas Radiol 1995; 39(4): 343-9.
[http://dx.doi.org/10.1111/j.1440-1673.1995.tb00309.x]

[46]   Pacella CM, Guglielmi R, Fabbrini R, *et al.* Papillary carcinoma in small hypoechoic thyroid nodules: predictive value of echo color Doppler evaluation Preliminary results Journal of experimental & clinical cancer research : CR 1998; 17(1): 127-8. Epub 1998/07/01

[47]   Iannuccilli JD, Cronan JJ, Monchik JM. Risk for malignancy of thyroid nodules as assessed by sonographic criteria: the need for biopsy. J Ultrasound Med 2004; 23(11): 1455-64. [http://dx.doi.org/10.7863/jum.2004.23.11.1455]

[48]   Rago T, Vitti P, Chiovato L, *et al.* Role of conventional ultrasonography and color flow-doppler sonography in predicting malignancy in 'cold' thyroid nodules. Eur J Endocrinol 1998; 138(1): 41-6. [http://dx.doi.org/10.1530/eje.0.1380041]

[49]   Shimamoto K, Endo T, Ishigaki T, Sakuma S, Makino N. Thyroid nodules: evaluation with color Doppler ultrasonography. J Ultrasound Med 1993; 12(11): 673-8. [http://dx.doi.org/10.7863/jum.1993.12.11.673]

[50]   Wienke JR, Chong WK, Fielding JR, Zou KH, Mittelstaedt CA. Sonographic features of benign thyroid nodules: interobserver reliability and overlap with malignancy. J Ultrasound Med 2003; 22(10): 1027-31. [http://dx.doi.org/10.7863/jum.2003.22.10.1027]

[51]   Moon HJ, Kwak JY, Kim MJ, Son EJ, Kim EK. Can vascularity at power Doppler US help predict thyroid malignancy? Radiology 2010; 255(1): 260-9. [http://dx.doi.org/10.1148/radiol.09091284]

[52]   Cappelli C, Castellano M, Pirola I, *et al.* The predictive value of ultrasound findings in the management of thyroid nodules. QJM 2007; 100(1): 29-35. [http://dx.doi.org/10.1093/qjmed/hcl121]

[53]   Chammas MC, Gerhard R, de Oliveira IR, *et al.* Thyroid nodules: evaluation with power Doppler and duplex Doppler ultrasound. Otolaryngol Head Neck Surg 2005; 132(6): 874-82. [http://dx.doi.org/10.1016/j.otohns.2005.02.003]

[54]   Sun J, Cai J, Wang X. Real-time ultrasound elastography for differentiation of benign and malignant thyroid nodules: a meta-analysis. J Ultrasound Med 2014; 33(3): 495-502. [http://dx.doi.org/10.7863/ultra.33.3.495]

[55]   Bojunga J, Herrmann E, Meyer G, Weber S, Zeuzem S, Friedrich-Rust M. Real-time elastography for the differentiation of benign and malignant thyroid nodules: a meta-analysis. Thyroid 2010; 20(10): 1145-50. [http://dx.doi.org/10.1089/thy.2010.0079]

[56]   Azizi G, Keller J, Lewis M, Puett D, Rivenbark K, Malchoff C. Performance of elastography for the evaluation of thyroid nodules: a prospective study. Thyroid 2013; 23(6): 734-40. [http://dx.doi.org/10.1089/thy.2012.0227]

[57]   Dighe M, Kim J, Luo S, Kim Y. Utility of the ultrasound elastographic systolic thyroid stiffness index in reducing fine-needle aspirations. J Ultrasound Med 2010; 29(4): 565-74. [http://dx.doi.org/10.7863/jum.2010.29.4.565]

[58]   Rago T, Scutari M, Santini F, *et al.* Real-time elastosonography: useful tool for refining the presurgical diagnosis in thyroid nodules with indeterminate or nondiagnostic cytology. J Clin Endocrinol Metab 2010; 95(12): 5274-80. [http://dx.doi.org/10.1210/jc.2010-0901]

[59]   Park SH, Kim SJ, Kim EK, Kim MJ, Son EJ, Kwak JY. Interobserver agreement in assessing the sonographic and elastographic features of malignant thyroid nodules. AJR Am J Roentgenol 2009; 193(5): W416-23.[http://dx.doi.org/10.2214/AJR.09.2541]

[60]   Bonavita JA, Mayo J, Babb J, *et al.* Pattern recognition of benign nodules at ultrasound of the thyroid: which nodules can be left alone? AJR Am J Roentgenol 2009; 193(1): 207-13. [http://dx.doi.org/10.2214/AJR.08.1820]

[61]   Hoang JK, Lee WK, Lee M, Johnson D, Farrell S US. Features of thyroid malignancy: pearls and pitfalls Radiographics : a review publication of the Radiological Society of North America, Inc 2007; 27(3): 847-60. Epub 2007/05/15

[62]   Lu C, Chang TC, Hsiao YL, Kuo MS. Ultrasonographic findings of papillary thyroid carcinoma and their relation to pathologic changes Journal of the Formosan Medical Association = Taiwan yi zhi 1994; 93(11-12): 933-8.

[63]   Propper RA, Skolnick ML, Weinstein BJ, Dekker A. The nonspecificity of the thyroid halo sign. J Clin Ultrasound 1980; 8(2): 129-32.
[http://dx.doi.org/10.1002/jcu.1870080206]

[64]   Yoon SJ, Yoon DY, Chang SK, *et al.* "Taller-than-wide sign" of thyroid malignancy: comparison between ultrasound and CT. AJR Am J Roentgenol 2010; 194(5): W420-4.
[http://dx.doi.org/10.2214/AJR.09.3376]

[65]   Reading CC, Charboneau JW, Hay ID, Sebo TJ. Sonography of thyroid nodules: a "classic pattern" diagnostic approach. Ultrasound Q 2005; 21(3): 157-65.
[http://dx.doi.org/10.1097/01.ruq.0000174750.27010.68]

[66]   Na DG, Baek JH, Sung JY, *et al.* Thyroid Imaging Reporting and Data System Risk Stratification of Thyroid Nodules: Categorization Based on Solidity and Echogenicity. Thyroid 2016; 26(4): 562-72.
[http://dx.doi.org/10.1089/thy.2015.0460]

[67]   Henrichsen TL, Reading CC, Charboneau JW, Donovan DJ, Sebo TJ, Hay ID. Cystic change in thyroid carcinoma: Prevalence and estimated volume in 360 carcinomas. J Clin Ultrasound 2010; 38(7): 361-6.

[68]   Kim DW, Lee EJ, In HS, Kim SJ. Sonographic differentiation of partially cystic thyroid nodules: a prospective study. AJNR Am J Neuroradiol 2010; 31(10): 1961-6.
[http://dx.doi.org/10.3174/ajnr.A2204]

[69]   Kwak JY, Kim EK, Youk JH, *et al.* Extrathyroid extension of well-differentiated papillary thyroid microcarcinoma on US. Thyroid 2008; 18(6): 609-14.
[http://dx.doi.org/10.1089/thy.2007.0345]

[70]   Lee CY, Kim SJ, Ko KR, Chung KW, Lee JH. Predictive factors for extrathyroidal extension of papillary thyroid carcinoma based on preoperative sonography. J Ultrasound Med 2014; 33(2): 231-8.
[http://dx.doi.org/10.7863/ultra.33.2.231]

[71]   Moon SJ, Kim DW, Kim SJ, Ha TK, Park HK, Jung SJ. Ultrasound assessment of degrees of extrathyroidal extension in papillary thyroid microcarcinoma. Endocr Pract 2014; 20(10): 1037-43.
[http://dx.doi.org/10.4158/EP14016.OR]

[72]   Rim JH, Chong S, Ryu HS, Chung BM, Ahn HS. Feasibility Study of Ultrasonographic Criteria for Microscopic and Macroscopic Extra-Thyroidal Extension Based on Thyroid Capsular Continuity and Tumor Contour in Patients with Papillary Thyroid Carcinomas. Ultrasound Med Biol 2016; 42(10): 2391-400.
[http://dx.doi.org/10.1016/j.ultrasmedbio.2016.06.014]

[73]   Solbiati L, Volterrani L, Rizzatto G, *et al.* The thyroid gland with low uptake lesions: evaluation by ultrasound. Radiology 1985; 155(1): 187-91.
[http://dx.doi.org/10.1148/radiology.155.1.3883413]

[74]   Cheng SP, Lee JJ, Lin JL, Chuang SM, Chien MN, Liu CL. Characterization of thyroid nodules using the proposed thyroid imaging reporting and data system (TI-RADS). Head Neck 2013; 35(4): 541-7.
[http://dx.doi.org/10.1002/hed.22985]

[75]   Russ G, Royer B, Bigorgne C, Rouxel A, Bienvenu-Perrard M, Leenhardt L. Prospective evaluation of thyroid imaging reporting and data system on 4550 nodules with and without elastography. Eur J Endocrinol 2013; 168(5): 649-55.
[http://dx.doi.org/10.1530/EJE-12-0936]

[76]   Tessler FN, Middleton WD, Grant EG, *et al.* ACR Thyroid Imaging, Reporting and Data System (TI-RADS): White Paper of the ACR TI-RADS Committee. Journal of the American College of Radiology: JACR 2017; 14(5): 587-95.

[http://dx.doi.org/10.1016/j.jacr.2017.01.046]

[77] Middleton WD, Teefey SA, Reading CC, *et al.* Comparison of Performance Characteristics of American College of Radiology TI-RADS, Korean Society of Thyroid Radiology TIRADS, and American Thyroid Association Guidelines. AJR Am J Roentgenol 2018; 210(5): 1148-54.
[http://dx.doi.org/10.2214/AJR.17.18822]

[78] Brander AE, Viikinkoski VP, Nickels JI, Kivisaari LM. Importance of thyroid abnormalities detected at US screening: a 5-year follow-up. Radiology 2000; 215(3): 801-6.
[http://dx.doi.org/10.1148/radiology.215.3.r00jn07801]

[79] Kuma K, Matsuzuka F, Yokozawa T, Miyauchi A, Sugawara M. Fate of untreated benign thyroid nodules: results of long-term follow-up. World J Surg 1994; 18(4): 495-8.
[http://dx.doi.org/10.1007/BF00353745]

[80] Erdogan MF, Gursoy A, Erdogan G. Natural course of benign thyroid nodules in a moderately iodine-deficient area. Clin Endocrinol (Oxf) 2006; 65(6): 767-71.
[http://dx.doi.org/10.1111/j.1365-2265.2006.02664.x]

[81] Moon WJ, Baek JH, Jung SL, *et al.* Ultrasonography and the ultrasound-based management of thyroid nodules: consensus statement and recommendations. Korean J Radiol 2011; 12(1): 1-14.
[http://dx.doi.org/10.3348/kjr.2011.12.1.1]

[82] McCoy KL, Jabbour N, Ogilvie JB, Ohori NP, Carty SE, Yim JH. The incidence of cancer and rate of false-negative cytology in thyroid nodules greater than or equal to 4 cm in size Surgery 2007; 142(6): 837-44.

[83] Porterfield JR Jr, Grant CS, Dean DS, *et al.* Reliability of benign fine needle aspiration cytology of large thyroid nodules. Surgery 2008; 144(6): 963-8.
[http://dx.doi.org/10.1016/j.surg.2008.09.006]

[84] Lew JI, Solorzano CC. Use of ultrasound in the management of thyroid cancer. Oncologist 2010; 15(3): 253-8.
[http://dx.doi.org/10.1634/theoncologist.2009-0324]

[85] Ying M, Ahuja A, Brook F. Sonographic appearances of cervical lymph nodes: variations by age and sex. J Clin Ultrasound 2002; 30(1): 1-11.
[http://dx.doi.org/10.1002/jcu.10022]

[86] Leenhardt L, Erdogan MF, Hegedus L, *et al.* 2013 European thyroid association guidelines for cervical ultrasound scan and ultrasound-guided techniques in the postoperative management of patients with thyroid cancer. Eur Thyroid J 2013; 2(3): 147-59.
[http://dx.doi.org/10.1159/000354537]

[87] Moreno MA, Agarwal G, de Luna R, *et al.* Preoperative lateral neck ultrasonography as a long-term outcome predictor in papillary thyroid cancer. Arch Otolaryngol Head Neck Surg 2011; 137(2): 157-62.
[http://dx.doi.org/10.1001/archoto.2010.254]

[88] Shimamoto K, Satake H, Sawaki A, Ishigaki T, Funahashi H, Imai T. Preoperative staging of thyroid papillary carcinoma with ultrasonography. Eur J Radiol 1998; 29(1): 4-10.
[http://dx.doi.org/10.1016/S0720-048X(97)00184-8]

[89] Solorzano CC, Carneiro DM, Ramirez M, Lee TM, Irvin GL III. Surgeon-performed ultrasound in the management of thyroid malignancy. Am Surg 2004; 70(7): 576-80.

[90] Machens A, Hinze R, Thomusch O, Dralle H. Pattern of nodal metastasis for primary and reoperative thyroid cancer. World J Surg 2002; 26(1): 22-8.
[http://dx.doi.org/10.1007/s00268-001-0176-3]

[91] Leboulleux S, Girard E, Rose M, *et al.* Ultrasound criteria of malignancy for cervical lymph nodes in patients followed up for differentiated thyroid cancer. J Clin Endocrinol Metab 2007; 92(9): 3590-4.
[http://dx.doi.org/10.1210/jc.2007-0444]

[92]   Kouvaraki MA, Shapiro SE, Fornage BD, *et al*. Role of preoperative ultrasonography in the surgical management of patients with thyroid cancer. Surgery 2003; 134(6): 946-54.
[http://dx.doi.org/10.1016/S0039-6060(03)00424-0]

[93]   Chow SM, Law SC, Chan JK, Au SK, Yau S, Lau WH. Papillary microcarcinoma of the thyroid-Prognostic significance of lymph node metastasis and multifocality. Cancer 2003; 98(1): 31-40.
[http://dx.doi.org/10.1002/cncr.11442]

[94]   Jeong HS, Baek CH, Son YI, *et al*. Integrated 18F-FDG PET/CT for the initial evaluation of cervical node level of patients with papillary thyroid carcinoma: comparison with ultrasound and contrast-enhanced CT. Clin Endocrinol (Oxf) 2006; 65(3): 402-7.
[http://dx.doi.org/10.1111/j.1365-2265.2006.02612.x]

[95]   Moreno MA, Edeiken-Monroe BS, Siegel ER, Sherman SI, Clayman GL. In papillary thyroid cancer, preoperative central neck ultrasound detects only macroscopic surgical disease, but negative findings predict excellent long-term regional control and survival. Thyroid 2012; 22(4): 347-55.
[http://dx.doi.org/10.1089/thy.2011.0121]

[96]   Kuna SK, Bracic I, Tesic V, Kuna K, Herceg GH, Dodig D. Ultrasonographic differentiation of benign from malignant neck lymphadenopathy in thyroid cancer. J Ultrasound Med 2006; 25(12): 1531-7.
[http://dx.doi.org/10.7863/jum.2006.25.12.1531]

[97]   Sohn YM, Kwak JY, Kim EK, Moon HJ, Kim SJ, Kim MJ. Diagnostic approach for evaluation of lymph node metastasis from thyroid cancer using ultrasound and fine-needle aspiration biopsy. AJR Am J Roentgenol 2010; 194(1): 38-43.
[http://dx.doi.org/10.2214/AJR.09.3128]

[98]   Sofferman RA. Interpretation of ultrasound Otolaryngologic clinics of North America 2010; 43(6): 1171-202. v-vi. Epub 2010/11/04
[http://dx.doi.org/10.1016/j.otc.2010.08.008]

[99]   Steinkamp HJ, Cornehl M, Hosten N, Pegios W, Vogl T, Felix R. Cervical lymphadenopathy: ratio of long- to short-axis diameter as a predictor of malignancy. Br J Radiol 1995; 68(807): 266-70.
[http://dx.doi.org/10.1259/0007-1285-68-807-266]

[100]   do Rosario PW, Fagundes TA, Maia FF, Franco AC, Figueiredo MB, Purisch S. Sonography in the diagnosis of cervical recurrence in patients with differentiated thyroid carcinoma. J Ultrasound Med 2004; 23(7): 915-20.
[http://dx.doi.org/10.7863/jum.2004.23.7.915]

[101]   Alam F, Naito K, Horiguchi J, Fukuda H, Tachikake T, Ito K. Accuracy of sonographic elastography in the differential diagnosis of enlarged cervical lymph nodes: comparison with conventional B-mode sonography. AJR Am J Roentgenol 2008; 191(2): 604-10.
[http://dx.doi.org/10.2214/AJR.07.3401]

[102]   Gharib H, Goellner JR. Fine-needle aspiration biopsy of the thyroid: an appraisal. Ann Intern Med 1993; 118(4): 282-9.
[http://dx.doi.org/10.7326/0003-4819-118-4-199302150-00007]

[103]   Hamberger B, Gharib H, Melton LJ III, Goellner JR, Zinsmeister AR. Fine-needle aspiration biopsy of thyroid nodules. Impact on thyroid practice and cost of care. Am J Med 1982; 73(3): 381-4.
[http://dx.doi.org/10.1016/0002-9343(82)90731-8]

[104]   Sebo TJ. What are the keys to successful thyroid FNA interpretation? Clin Endocrinol (Oxf) 2012; 77(1): 13-7.
[http://dx.doi.org/10.1111/j.1365-2265.2012.04404.x]

[105]   Danese D, Sciacchitano S, Farsetti A, Andreoli M, Pontecorvi A. Diagnostic accuracy of conventional *versus* sonography-guided fine-needle aspiration biopsy of thyroid nodules. Thyroid 1998; 8(1): 15-21.
[http://dx.doi.org/10.1089/thy.1998.8.15]

[106]   Takashima S, Fukuda H, Kobayashi T. Thyroid nodules: clinical effect of ultrasound-guided fine-

needle aspiration biopsy. J Clin Ultrasound 1994; 22(9): 535-42.
[http://dx.doi.org/10.1002/jcu.1870220904]

[107] Baskin HJ. Ultrasound-guided fine-needle aspiration biopsy of thyroid nodules and multinodular goiters. Endocr Pract 2004; 10(3): 242-5.
[http://dx.doi.org/10.4158/EP.10.3.242]

[108] Ceresini G, Corcione L, Morganti S, *et al.* Ultrasound-guided fine-needle capillary biopsy of thyroid nodules, coupled with on-site cytologic review, improves results. Thyroid 2004; 14(5): 385-9.
[http://dx.doi.org/10.1089/105072504774193230]

[109] de Carvalho GA, Paz-Filho G, Cavalcanti TC, Graf H. Adequacy and diagnostic accuracy of aspiration *vs.* capillary fine needle thyroid biopsies. Endocr Pathol 2009; 20(4): 204-8.
[http://dx.doi.org/10.1007/s12022-009-9092-0]

[110] Moss WJ, Finegersh A, Pang J, *et al.* Needle Biopsy of Routine Thyroid Nodules Should Be Performed Using a Capillary Action Technique with 24- to 27-Gauge Needles: A Systematic Review and Meta-Analysis. Thyroid 2018; 28(7): 857-63.
[http://dx.doi.org/10.1089/thy.2017.0643]

[111] Gharib H, Papini E, Garber JR, *et al.* American Association of Clinical Endocrinologists, American College of Endocrinology, and Associazione Medici Endocrinologi Medical Guidelines for Clinical Practice for the Diagnosis and Management of Thyroid Nodules--2016 Update. Endocr Pract 2016; 22(5): 622-39.

[112] Abu-Yousef MM, Larson JH, Kuehn DM, Wu AS, Laroia AT. Safety of ultrasound-guided fine needle aspiration biopsy of neck lesions in patients taking antithrombotic/anticoagulant medications. Ultrasound Q 2011; 27(3): 157-9.
[http://dx.doi.org/10.1097/RUQ.0b013e31822b5681]

[113] Pena JM, Arnold J. Thyroid Fine Needle Aspiration Smear Preparation VideoEndocrinology 2017.[http://dx.doi.org/101089/ve20170097]

[114] Dean DS, Gharib H. Fine-Needle Aspiration Biopsy of the Thyroid Gland in: Endotext [Internet] South Dartmouth (MA): MDTextcom, Inc. 2000. 2000, Updated 2015 Apr 26, Cited 2018 Sept 22 [cited 2018 22 Sept]. Available from: https://www.ncbi.nlm.nih.gov/books/NBK285544/

[115] Duncan LD, Forrest L, Law WM Jr, Hubbard E, Stewart LE. Evaluation of thyroid fine-needle aspirations: can ThinPrep be used exclusively to appropriately triage patients having a thyroid nodule? Diagn Cytopathol 2011; 39(5): 341-8.
[http://dx.doi.org/10.1002/dc.21392]

[116] Fadda G, Rossi ED. Liquid-based cytology in fine-needle aspiration biopsies of the thyroid gland. Acta Cytol 2011; 55(5): 389-400.
[http://dx.doi.org/10.1159/000329029]

[117] Adeniran AJ, Theoharis C, Hui P, *et al.* Reflex BRAF testing in thyroid fine-needle aspiration biopsy with equivocal and positive interpretation: a prospective study. Thyroid 2011; 21(7): 717-23.
[http://dx.doi.org/10.1089/thy.2011.0021]

[118] Ferrari SM, Fallahi P, Ruffilli I, *et al.* Molecular testing in the diagnosis of differentiated thyroid carcinomas. Gland Surg 2018; 7 (Suppl. 1): S19-29.
[http://dx.doi.org/10.21037/gs.2017.11.07]

[119] Diazzi C, Madeo B, Taliani E, *et al.* The diagnostic value of calcitonin measurement in wash-out fluid from fine-needle aspiration of thyroid nodules in the diagnosis of medullary thyroid cancer. Endocr Pract 2013; 19(5): 769-79.
[http://dx.doi.org/10.4158/EP12420.OR]

[120] Kudo T, Miyauchi A, Ito Y, Takamura Y, Amino N, Hirokawa M. Diagnosis of medullary thyroid carcinoma by calcitonin measurement in fine-needle aspiration biopsy specimens. Thyroid 2007; 17(7): 635-8.

[http://dx.doi.org/10.1089/thy.2006.0338]

[121] Boi F, Maurelli I, Pinna G, *et al.* Calcitonin measurement in wash-out fluid from fine needle aspiration of neck masses in patients with primary and metastatic medullary thyroid carcinoma. J Clin Endocrinol Metab 2007; 92(6): 2115-8.
[http://dx.doi.org/10.1210/jc.2007-0326]

[122] Agarwal AM, Bentz JS, Hungerford R, Abraham D. Parathyroid fine-needle aspiration cytology in the evaluation of parathyroid adenoma: cytologic findings from 53 patients. Diagn Cytopathol 2009; 37(6): 407-10.
[http://dx.doi.org/10.1002/dc.21020]

[123] Crippa S, Mazzucchelli L, Cibas ES, Ali SZ. The Bethesda System for reporting thyroid fine-needle aspiration specimens. Am J Clin Pathol 2010; 134(2): 343-4.
[http://dx.doi.org/10.1309/AJCPXM9WIRQ8JZBJ]

[124] Cibas ES, Ali SZ. The 2017 Bethesda System for Reporting Thyroid Cytopathology. Thyroid 2017; 27(11): 1341-6.
[http://dx.doi.org/10.1089/thy.2017.0500]

[125] Bongiovanni M, Spitale A, Faquin WC, Mazzucchelli L, Baloch ZW. The Bethesda System for Reporting Thyroid Cytopathology: a meta-analysis. Acta Cytol 2012; 56(4): 333-9.
[http://dx.doi.org/10.1159/000339959]

[126] Hirsch D, Robenshtok E, Bachar G, Braslavsky D, Benbassat C. The Implementation of the Bethesda System for Reporting Thyroid Cytopathology Improves Malignancy Detection Despite Lower Rate of Thyroidectomy in Indeterminate Nodules. World J Surg 2015; 39(8): 1959-65.
[http://dx.doi.org/10.1007/s00268-015-3032-6]

[127] Moon HJ, Kwak JY, Choi YS, Kim EK. How to manage thyroid nodules with two consecutive non-diagnostic results on ultrasonography-guided fine-needle aspiration. World J Surg 2012; 36(3): 586-92.
[http://dx.doi.org/10.1007/s00268-011-1397-8]

[128] Layfield LJ, Abrams J, Cochand-Priollet B, *et al.* Post-thyroid FNA testing and treatment options: a synopsis of the National Cancer Institute Thyroid Fine Needle Aspiration State of the Science Conference. Diagn Cytopathol 2008; 36(6): 442-8.
[http://dx.doi.org/10.1002/dc.20832]

[129] Lubitz CC, Nagarkatti S, Faquin WC, *et al.* Diagnostic Yield of Repeat Fine-Needle Aspiration For Non-Diagnostic Thyroid Nodule Biopsy Is Not Altered by Timing. Thyroid 2012.

[130] Singh RS, Wang HH. Timing of repeat thyroid fine-needle aspiration in the management of thyroid nodules. Acta Cytol 2011; 55(6): 544-8.
[http://dx.doi.org/10.1159/000334214]

[131] Alexander EK, Heering JP, Benson CB, *et al.* Assessment of nondiagnostic ultrasound-guided fine needle aspirations of thyroid nodules. J Clin Endocrinol Metab 2002; 87(11): 4924-7.
[http://dx.doi.org/10.1210/jc.2002-020865]

[132] Choi YS, Hong SW, Kwak JY, Moon HJ, Kim EK. Clinical and ultrasonographic findings affecting nondiagnostic results upon the second fine needle aspiration for thyroid nodules. Ann Surg Oncol 2012; 19(7): 2304-9.
[http://dx.doi.org/10.1245/s10434-012-2288-4]

[133] Renshaw AA, Pinnar N. Comparison of thyroid fine-needle aspiration and core needle biopsy. Am J Clin Pathol 2007; 128(3): 370-4.
[http://dx.doi.org/10.1309/07TL3V58337TXHMC]

[134] Yeon JS, Baek JH, Lim HK, *et al.* Thyroid nodules with initially nondiagnostic cytologic results: the role of core-needle biopsy. Radiology 2013; 268(1): 274-80.
[http://dx.doi.org/10.1148/radiol.13122247]

[135] Kwak JY, Koo H, Youk JH, *et al.* Value of US correlation of a thyroid nodule with initially benign cytologic results. Radiology 2010; 254(1): 292-300.
[http://dx.doi.org/10.1148/radiol.2541090460]

[136] Oertel YC, Miyahara-Felipe L, Mendoza MG, Yu K. Value of repeated fine needle aspirations of the thyroid: an analysis of over ten thousand FNAs. Thyroid 2007; 17(11): 1061-6.
[http://dx.doi.org/10.1089/thy.2007.0159]

[137] Illouz F, Rodien P, Saint-Andre JP, *et al.* Usefulness of repeated fine-needle cytology in the follow-up of non-operated thyroid nodules. Eur J Endocrinol 2007; 156(3): 303-8.
[http://dx.doi.org/10.1530/EJE-06-0616]

[138] Kuru B, Gulcelik NE, Gulcelik MA, Dincer H. The false-negative rate of fine-needle aspiration cytology for diagnosing thyroid carcinoma in thyroid nodules. Langenbecks Arch Surg 2010; 395(2): 127-32.
[http://dx.doi.org/10.1007/s00423-009-0470-3]

[139] Pinchot SN, Al-Wagih H, Schaefer S, Sippel R, Chen H. Accuracy of fine-needle aspiration biopsy for predicting neoplasm or carcinoma in thyroid nodules 4 cm or larger. Arch Surg 2009; 144(7): 649-55.
[http://dx.doi.org/10.1001/archsurg.2009.116]

[140] Wharry LI, McCoy KL, Stang MT, *et al.* Thyroid nodules (>/=4 cm): can ultrasound and cytology reliably exclude cancer? World J Surg 2014; 38(3): 614-21.
[http://dx.doi.org/10.1007/s00268-013-2261-9]

[141] Yoon JH, Kwak JY, Moon HJ, Kim MJ, Kim EK. The diagnostic accuracy of ultrasound-guided fine-needle aspiration biopsy and the sonographic differences between benign and malignant thyroid nodules 3 cm or larger. Thyroid 2011; 21(9): 993-1000.
[http://dx.doi.org/10.1089/thy.2010.0458]

[142] Yoo WS, Choi HS, Cho SW, *et al.* The role of ultrasound findings in the management of thyroid nodules with atypia or follicular lesions of undetermined significance. Clin Endocrinol (Oxf) 2014; 80(5): 735-42.
[http://dx.doi.org/10.1111/cen.12348]

[143] Gweon HM, Son EJ, Youk JH, Kim JA. Thyroid nodules with Bethesda system III cytology: can ultrasonography guide the next step? Ann Surg Oncol 2013; 20(9): 3083-8.
[http://dx.doi.org/10.1245/s10434-013-2990-x]

[144] Baloch Z. Role of repeat fine-needle aspiration biopsy (FNAB) in the management of thyroid nodules. Diagn Cytopathol 2003; 29(4): 203-6.
[http://dx.doi.org/10.1002/dc.10361]

[145] Nayar R, Ivanovic M. The indeterminate thyroid fine-needle aspiration: experience from an academic center using terminology similar to that proposed in the 2007 National Cancer Institute Thyroid Fine Needle Aspiration State of the Science Conference. Cancer 2009; 117(3): 195-202.

[146] VanderLaan PA, Marqusee E, Krane JF. Clinical outcome for atypia of undetermined significance in thyroid fine-needle aspirations: should repeated fna be the preferred initial approach? Am J Clin Pathol 2011; 135(5): 770-5.
[http://dx.doi.org/10.1309/AJCP4P2GCCDNHFMY]

[147] Na DG, Kim JH, Sung JY, *et al.* Core-needle biopsy is more useful than repeat fine-needle aspiration in thyroid nodules read as nondiagnostic or atypia of undetermined significance by the Bethesda system for reporting thyroid cytopathology. Thyroid 2012; 22(5): 468-75.
[http://dx.doi.org/10.1089/thy.2011.0185]

[148] Rosario PW, Purisch S. Ultrasonographic characteristics as a criterion for repeat cytology in benign thyroid nodules. Arq Bras Endocrinol Metabol 2010; 54(1): 52-5.
[http://dx.doi.org/10.1590/S0004-27302010000100009]

[149] Singh Ospina N, Maraka S, Espinosa DeYcaza A, *et al.* Diagnostic accuracy of thyroid nodule growth

to predict malignancy in thyroid nodules with benign cytology: systematic review and meta-analysis. Clin Endocrinol (Oxf) 2016; 85(1): 122-31.
[http://dx.doi.org/10.1111/cen.12975]

[150] Durante C, Costante G, Lucisano G, *et al.* The natural history of benign thyroid nodules. JAMA 2015; 313(9): 926-35.
[http://dx.doi.org/10.1001/jama.2015.0956]

[151] Pacini F, Molinaro E, Castagna MG, *et al.* Recombinant human thyrotropin-stimulated serum thyroglobulin combined with neck ultrasonography has the highest sensitivity in monitoring differentiated thyroid carcinoma. J Clin Endocrinol Metab 2003; 88(8): 3668-73.
[http://dx.doi.org/10.1210/jc.2002-021925]

[152] Torlontano M, Attard M, Crocetti U, *et al.* Follow-up of low risk patients with papillary thyroid cancer: role of neck ultrasonography in detecting lymph node metastases. J Clin Endocrinol Metab 2004; 89(7): 3402-7.
[http://dx.doi.org/10.1210/jc.2003-031521]

[153] Frasoldati A, Pesenti M, Gallo M, Caroggio A, Salvo D, Valcavi R. Diagnosis of neck recurrences in patients with differentiated thyroid carcinoma. Cancer 2003; 97(1): 90-6.
[http://dx.doi.org/10.1002/cncr.11031]

[154] Rouxel A, Hejblum G, Bernier MO, *et al.* Prognostic factors associated with the survival of patients developing loco-regional recurrences of differentiated thyroid carcinomas. J Clin Endocrinol Metab 2004; 89(11): 5362-8.
[http://dx.doi.org/10.1210/jc.2003-032004]

[155] Schlumberger MJ. Papillary and follicular thyroid carcinoma. N Engl J Med 1998; 338(5): 297-306.
[http://dx.doi.org/10.1056/NEJM199801293380506]

[156] Chua WY, Langer JE, Jones LP. Surveillance Neck Sonography After Thyroidectomy for Papillary Thyroid Carcinoma: Pitfalls in the Diagnosis of Locally Recurrent and Metastatic Disease. J Ultrasound Med 2017; 36(7): 1511-30.
[http://dx.doi.org/10.7863/ultra.16.08086]

[157] Ko MS, Lee JH, Shong YK, Gong GY, Baek JH. Normal and abnormal sonographic findings at the thyroidectomy sites in postoperative patients with thyroid malignancy. AJR Am J Roentgenol 2010; 194(6): 1596-609.
[http://dx.doi.org/10.2214/AJR.09.2513]

[158] Kamaya A, Gross M, Akatsu H, Jeffrey RB. Recurrence in the thyroidectomy bed: sonographic findings. AJR Am J Roentgenol 2011; 196(1): 66-70.
[http://dx.doi.org/10.2214/AJR.10.4474]

[159] Shin JH, Han BK, Ko EY, Kang SS. Sonographic findings in the surgical bed after thyroidectomy: comparison of recurrent tumors and nonrecurrent lesions. J Ultrasound Med 2007; 26(10): 1359-66.
[http://dx.doi.org/10.7863/jum.2007.26.10.1359]

[160] Kobayashi K, Hirokawa M, Yabuta T, *et al.* Tumor thrombus of thyroid malignancies in veins: importance of detection by ultrasonography. Thyroid 2011; 21(5): 527-31.
[http://dx.doi.org/10.1089/thy.2010.0099]

[161] Marcy PY, Thariat J, Bozec A, Poissonnet G, Benisvy D, Dassonville O. Venous obstruction of thyroid malignancy origin: the Antoine Lacassagne Institute experience. World J Surg Oncol 2009; 7: 40.[http://dx.doi.org/10.1186/1477-7819-7-40]

[162] Pacini F, Fugazzola L, Lippi F, *et al.* Detection of thyroglobulin in fine needle aspirates of nonthyroidal neck masses: a clue to the diagnosis of metastatic differentiated thyroid cancer. J Clin Endocrinol Metab 1992; 74(6): 1401-4.

[163] Boi F, Baghino G, Atzeni F, Lai ML, Faa G, Mariotti S. The diagnostic value for differentiated thyroid carcinoma metastases of thyroglobulin (Tg) measurement in washout fluid from fine-needle aspiration

biopsy of neck lymph nodes is maintained in the presence of circulating anti-Tg antibodies. J Clin Endocrinol Metab 2006; 91(4): 1364-9.
[http://dx.doi.org/10.1210/jc.2005-1705]

[164] Cunha N, Rodrigues F, Curado F, *et al.* Thyroglobulin detection in fine-needle aspirates of cervical lymph nodes: a technique for the diagnosis of metastatic differentiated thyroid cancer. Eur J Endocrinol 2007; 157(1): 101-7.
[http://dx.doi.org/10.1530/EJE-07-0088]

[165] Giovanella L, Bongiovanni M, Trimboli P. Diagnostic value of thyroglobulin assay in cervical lymph node fine-needle aspirations for metastatic differentiated thyroid cancer. Curr Opin Oncol 2013; 25(1): 6-13.
[http://dx.doi.org/10.1097/CCO.0b013e32835a9ab1]

[166] Borel AL, Boizel R, Faure P, *et al.* Significance of low levels of thyroglobulin in fine needle aspirates from cervical lymph nodes of patients with a history of differentiated thyroid cancer. Eur J Endocrinol 2008; 158(5): 691-8.
[http://dx.doi.org/10.1530/EJE-07-0749]

[167] Moon JH, Kim YI, Lim JA, *et al.* Thyroglobulin in Washout Fluid From Lymph Node Fine-needle Aspiration Biopsy in Papillary Thyroid Cancer: Large-scale Validation of the Cutoff Value to Determine Malignancy and Evaluation of Discrepant Results. J Clin Endocrinol Metab 2013; 98(3): 1061-8.
[http://dx.doi.org/10.1210/jc.2012-3291]

[168] Jeon MJ, Park JW, Han JM, *et al.* Serum antithyroglobulin antibodies interfere with thyroglobulin detection in fine-needle aspirates of metastatic neck nodes in papillary thyroid carcinoma. J Clin Endocrinol Metab 2013; 98(1): 153-60.
[http://dx.doi.org/10.1210/jc.2012-2369]

[169] McCoy KL, Yim JH, Tublin ME, Burmeister LA, Ogilvie JB, Carty SE. Same-day ultrasound guidance in reoperation for locally recurrent papillary thyroid cancer. Surgery 2007; 142(6): 965-72.
[http://dx.doi.org/10.1016/j.surg.2007.09.021]

[170] Harari A, Sippel RS, Goldstein R, *et al.* Successful localization of recurrent thyroid cancer in reoperative neck surgery using ultrasound-guided methylene blue dye injection. J Am Coll Surg 2012; 215(4): 555-61.
[http://dx.doi.org/10.1016/j.jamcollsurg.2012.06.006]

[171] Robenshtok E, Fish S, Bach A, Dominguez JM, Shaha A, Tuttle RM. Suspicious cervical lymph nodes detected after thyroidectomy for papillary thyroid cancer usually remain stable over years in properly selected patients. J Clin Endocrinol Metab 2012; 97(8): 2706-13.
[http://dx.doi.org/10.1210/jc.2012-1553]

[172] Al-Saif O, Farrar WB, Bloomston M, Porter K, Ringel MD, Kloos RT. Long-term efficacy of lymph node reoperation for persistent papillary thyroid cancer. J Clin Endocrinol Metab 2010; 95(5): 2187-94.
[http://dx.doi.org/10.1210/jc.2010-0063]

[173] Mazziotti G, Sorvillo F, Iorio S, *et al.* Grey-scale analysis allows a quantitative evaluation of thyroid echogenicity in the patients with Hashimoto's thyroiditis. Clin Endocrinol (Oxf) 2003; 59(2): 223-9.
[http://dx.doi.org/10.1046/j.1365-2265.2003.01829.x]

[174] Loy M, Cianchetti ME, Cardia F, Melis A, Boi F, Mariotti S. Correlation of computerized gray-scale sonographic findings with thyroid function and thyroid autoimmune activity in patients with Hashimoto's thyroiditis. J Clin Ultrasound 2004; 32(3): 136-40.
[http://dx.doi.org/10.1002/jcu.20008]

[175] Rotondi M, Cappelli C, Leporati P, *et al.* A hypoechoic pattern of the thyroid at ultrasound does not indicate autoimmune thyroid diseases in patients with morbid obesity. Eur J Endocrinol 2010; 163(1): 105-9.

[http://dx.doi.org/10.1530/EJE-10-0288]

[176] Yeh HC, Futterweit W, Gilbert P. Micronodulation: ultrasonographic sign of Hashimoto thyroiditis. J Ultrasound Med 1996; 15(12): 813-9.
[http://dx.doi.org/10.7863/jum.1996.15.12.813]

[177] Vitti P, Rago T, Mancusi F, *et al.* Thyroid hypoechogenic pattern at ultrasonography as a tool for predicting recurrence of hyperthyroidism after medical treatment in patients with Graves' disease. Acta Endocrinol (Copenh) 1992; 126(2): 128-31.
[http://dx.doi.org/10.1530/acta.0.1260128]

[178] Saleh A, Cohnen M, Furst G, Modder U, Feldkamp J. Prediction of relapse after antithyroid drug therapy of Graves' disease: value of color Doppler sonography. Exp Clin Endocrinol Diabetes 2004; 112(9): 510-3.
[http://dx.doi.org/10.1055/s-2004-821308]

[179] Varsamidis K, Varsamidou E, Mavropoulos G. Doppler ultrasonography in predicting relapse of hyperthyroidism in Graves' disease. Acta Radiol 2000; 41(1): 45-8.
[http://dx.doi.org/10.1258/rsmacta.41.1.45]

[180] Belfiore A, Russo D, Vigneri R, Filetti S. Graves' disease, thyroid nodules and thyroid cancer. Clin Endocrinol (Oxf) 2001; 55(6): 711-8.
[http://dx.doi.org/10.1046/j.1365-2265.2001.01415.x]

[181] Stocker DJ, Burch HB. Thyroid cancer yield in patients with Graves' disease. Minerva Endocrinol 2003; 28(3): 205-12.

[182] Johnson NA, Carty SE, Tublin ME. Parathyroid imaging Radiol Clin North Am 2011; 49(3): 489-509. vi. Epub 2011/05/17
[http://dx.doi.org/10.1016/j.rcl.2011.02.009]

[183] Gilmour JR. The embryology of the parathyroid glands, the thymus and certain associated rudiments. J Pathol 1937; 45: 507.[http://dx.doi.org/10.1002/path.1700450304]

[184] Wang C. The anatomic basis of parathyroid surgery. Ann Surg 1976; 183(3): 271-5.
[http://dx.doi.org/10.1097/00000658-197603000-00010]

[185] Akerstrom G, Malmaeus J, Bergstrom R. Surgical anatomy of human parathyroid glands. Surgery 1984; 95(1): 14-21.

[186] Yip L, Pryma DA, Yim JH, Virji MA, Carty SE, Ogilvie JB. Can a lightbulb sestamibi SPECT accurately predict single-gland disease in sporadic primary hyperparathyroidism? World J Surg 2008; 32(5): 784-92.
[http://dx.doi.org/10.1007/s00268-008-9532-x]

[187] Carty SE, Worsey J, Virji MA, Brown ML, Watson CG. Concise parathyroidectomy: the impact of preoperative SPECT 99mTc sestamibi scanning and intraoperative quick parathormone assay. Surgery 1997; 122(6): 1107-14.
[http://dx.doi.org/10.1016/S0039-6060(97)90215-4]

[188] Siperstein A, Berber E, Mackey R, Alghoul M, Wagner K, Milas M. Prospective evaluation of sestamibi scan, ultrasonography, and rapid PTH to predict the success of limited exploration for sporadic primary hyperparathyroidism. Surgery 2004; 136(4): 872-80.
[http://dx.doi.org/10.1016/j.surg.2004.06.024]

[189] Grimelius L, Bondeson L. Histopathological diagnosis of parathyroid diseases. Pathol Res Pract 1995; 191(4): 353-65.
[http://dx.doi.org/10.1016/S0344-0338(11)80889-7]

[190] Morita SY, Somervell H, Umbricht CB, Dackiw AP, Zeiger MA. Evaluation for concomitant thyroid nodules and primary hyperparathyroidism in patients undergoing parathyroidectomy or thyroidectomy. Surgery 2008; 144(6): 862-6.
[http://dx.doi.org/10.1016/j.surg.2008.07.029]

[191] Milas M, Mensah A, Alghoul M, *et al.* The impact of office neck ultrasonography on reducing unnecessary thyroid surgery in patients undergoing parathyroidectomy. Thyroid 2005; 15(9): 1055-9. [http://dx.doi.org/10.1089/thy.2005.15.1055]

[192] Adler JT, Chen H, Schaefer S, Sippel RS. Does routine use of ultrasound result in additional thyroid procedures in patients with primary hyperparathyroidism? J Am Coll Surg 2010; 211(4): 536-9. [http://dx.doi.org/10.1016/j.jamcollsurg.2010.05.015]

[193] Lee L, Steward DL. Techniques for parathyroid localization with ultrasound. Otolaryngol Clin North Am 2010; 43(6): 1229-39. [vi.]. [http://dx.doi.org/10.1016/j.otc.2010.08.002]

[194] Rickes S, Sitzy J, Neye H, Ocran KW, Wermke W. High-resolution ultrasound in combination with colour-Doppler sonography for preoperative localization of parathyroid adenomas in patients with primary hyperparathyroidism. Ultraschall Med 2003; 24(2): 85-9. [http://dx.doi.org/10.1055/s-2003-38667]

[195] Hara H, Igarashi A, Yano Y, *et al.* Ultrasonographic features of parathyroid carcinoma. Endocr J 2001; 48(2): 213-7. [http://dx.doi.org/10.1507/endocrj.48.213]

[196] Ruda JM, Hollenbeak CS, Stack BC Jr. A systematic review of the diagnosis and treatment of primary hyperparathyroidism from 1995 to 2003. Otolaryngol Head Neck Surg 2005; 132(3): 359-72. [http://dx.doi.org/10.1016/j.otohns.2004.10.005]

[197] Lumachi F, Zucchetta P, Marzola MC, *et al.* Advantages of combined technetium-99m-sestamibi scintigraphy and high-resolution ultrasonography in parathyroid localization: comparative study in 91 patients with primary hyperparathyroidism. Eur J Endocrinol 2000; 143(6): 755-60. [http://dx.doi.org/10.1530/eje.0.1430755]

[198] Solorzano CC, Carneiro-Pla DM, Irvin GL III. Surgeon-performed ultrasonography as the initial and only localizing study in sporadic primary hyperparathyroidism. J Am Coll Surg 2006; 202(1): 18-24. [http://dx.doi.org/10.1016/j.jamcollsurg.2005.08.014]

[199] Lal G, Clark OH. Primary hyperparathyroidism: controversies in surgical management. Trends in endocrinology and metabolism. TEM 2003; 14(9): 417-22.

[200] Sugg SL, Krzywda EA, Demeure MJ, Wilson SD. Detection of multiple gland primary hyperparathyroidism in the era of minimally invasive parathyroidectomy. Surgery 2004; 136(6): 1303-9. [http://dx.doi.org/10.1016/j.surg.2004.06.062]

[201] Rozman B. bence-Zigman Z, Tomic-Brzac H, Skreb F, Pavlinovic Z, Simonovic I. Sclerosation of thyroid cyst by ethanol. Period Biol 1989; 91: 1116-8.

[202] Baskin HJ. Percutaneous ethanol injection of thyroglossal duct cysts. Endocr Pract 2006; 12(4): 355-7. [http://dx.doi.org/10.4158/EP.12.4.355]

[203] Bennedbaek FN, Hegedus L. Treatment of recurrent thyroid cysts with ethanol: a randomized double-blind controlled trial. J Clin Endocrinol Metab 2003; 88(12): 5773-7. [http://dx.doi.org/10.1210/jc.2003-031000]

[204] Valcavi R, Frasoldati A. Ultrasound-guided percutaneous ethanol injection therapy in thyroid cystic nodules. Endocr Pract 2004; 10(3): 269-75. [http://dx.doi.org/10.4158/EP.10.3.269]

[205] Guglielmi R, Pacella CM, Bianchini A, *et al.* Percutaneous ethanol injection treatment in benign thyroid lesions: role and efficacy. Thyroid 2004; 14(2): 125-31. [http://dx.doi.org/10.1089/105072504322880364]

[206] Zieleznik W, Kawczyk-Krupka A, Barlik MP, Cebula W, Sieron A. Modified percutaneous ethanol injection in the treatment of viscous cystic thyroid nodules. Thyroid 2005; 15(7): 683-6.

[http://dx.doi.org/10.1089/thy.2005.15.683]

[207] Livraghi T, Paracchi A, Ferrari C, Reschini E, Macchi RM, Bonifacino A. Treatment of autonomous thyroid nodules with percutaneous ethanol injection: 4-year experience. Radiology 1994; 190(2): 529-33.
[http://dx.doi.org/10.1148/radiology.190.2.8284411]

[208] Veldman MW, Reading CC, Farrell MA, *et al*. Percutaneous parathyroid ethanol ablation in patients with multiple endocrine neoplasia type 1. AJR Am J Roentgenol 2008; 191(6): 1740-4.
[http://dx.doi.org/10.2214/AJR.07.3431]

[209] Heilo A, Sigstad E, Fagerlid KH, *et al*. Efficacy of ultrasound-guided percutaneous ethanol injection treatment in patients with a limited number of metastatic cervical lymph nodes from papillary thyroid carcinoma. J Clin Endocrinol Metab 2011; 96(9): 2750-5.
[http://dx.doi.org/10.1210/jc.2010-2952]

[210] Hay ID, Charboneau JW. The coming of age of ultrasound-guided percutaneous ethanol ablation of selected neck nodal metastases in well-differentiated thyroid carcinoma. J Clin Endocrinol Metab 2011; 96(9): 2717-20.
[http://dx.doi.org/10.1210/jc.2011-2196]

[211] Lewis BD, Hay ID, Charboneau JW, McIver B, Reading CC, Goellner JR. Percutaneous ethanol injection for treatment of cervical lymph node metastases in patients with papillary thyroid carcinoma. AJR Am J Roentgenol 2002; 178(3): 699-704.
[http://dx.doi.org/10.2214/ajr.178.3.1780699]

[212] Goletti O, Monzani F, Caraccio N, *et al*. Percutaneous ethanol injection treatment of autonomously functioning single thyroid nodules: optimization of treatment and short term outcome. World J Surg 1992; 16(4): 784-9.
[http://dx.doi.org/10.1007/BF02067387]

[213] Harman CR, Grant CS, Hay ID, *et al*. Indications, technique, and efficacy of alcohol injection of enlarged parathyroid glands in patients with primary hyperparathyroidism. Surgery 1998; 124(6): 1011-9.
[http://dx.doi.org/10.1067/msy.1998.91826]

[214] Bumpous JM, Randolph GW. The expanding utility of office-based ultrasound for the head and neck surgeon Otolaryngologic clinics of North America 2010; 43(6): 1203-8. vi. Epub 2010/11/04

LIST OF ABBREVIATIONS AND SYMBOLS

AACE	American Association of Clinical Endocrinologists
ACR	American College of Radiology
AIH	Amiodarone-induced hyperthyroidism
AITD	Autoimmune thyroid disease
AP	Anteroposterior
ATA	American Thyroid Association
AUS	Atypia of undetermined significance
BSRTC	Bethesda System for Reporting Thyroid Cytopathology
c	Propagation velocity
C	Carotid artery
cc	Cubic Centimeters
CCA	Common carotid artery
CLN	Cervical lymph node
CS	Carotid sheath
CSI	Compound spatial imaging
CT	Computed tomography
DIG	Anterior belly of the digastric muscle
DTC	Differentiated thyroid cancer
ESR	Erythrocyte sedimentation rate
ETA	European Thyroid Association
ETE	Extra-thyroidal extension
EU-TIRADS	European Thyroid Imaging Reporting and Data System
f	Frequency
FLUS	Follicular lesion of undetermined significance
FN	Follicular neoplasm
FNA	Fine needle aspiration
FNA-Tg	FNA-Thyroglobulin
FTC	Follicular thyroid cancer
GD	Graves' disease
HT	Hashimoto's thyroiditis

Hz	Hertz
IJV	Internal Jugular vein
INR	International normalized ratio
λ	Wavelength
LA	Long-axis
LC	Longus colli muscle
MEN	Multiple endocrine neoplasia
MHz	Megahertz
MNG	Multinodular goitre
MRI	Magnetic resonance imaging
MTC	Medullary thyroid cancer
NIFTP	Non-invasive follicular thyroid neoplasm with papillary-like nuclear features
NOAC	Novel oral anticoagulants
NPV	Negative predictive value
Oesoph	Oesophagus
p	Density of the medium
P	Parathyroid gland
PEI	Percutaneous ethanol injection
PET	Positron emission tomography
PPV	Positive predictive value
PTC	Papillary thyroid cancer
PTH	Parathyroid hormone
ROSE	Rapid on-site cytological evaluation
SA	Short-axis
SCM	Sternocleidomastoid muscle
SFN	Suspicious for follicular neoplasm
SM	Strap muscles of the neck
SPECT	Single photon emission tomography
SUSP	Suspicious for malignancy
TGD	Thyroglossal duct
THI	Tissue harmonic imaging
TI-RADS	Thyroid Imaging Reporting and Data System
TNM	Tumour, node, metastases

TPO-Ab	Anti-thyroid peroxidase antibodies
TSHR-Ab	Anti-TSH-receptor antibodies
TTW	Taller-than-wide
UG-FNA	Ultrasound-guided FNA
US	Ultrasound
USE	Ultrasound elastography
Z	Acoustic impedance

SUBJECT INDEX